Lady's Companion For

Menopause

Treated Naturally

Mark Gilberd
Homoeopath. Medical Herbalist and Iridologist

Index

Antiviral, Antiviral, Antirheumatic, Aperient, Astringent, Bitter, Carminative, Cardioactive, Cholagogue, Demulcent, Diaphoretic, Diuretic, Emmenagogue, Expectorant, Febrifuge, Galactagogue, Hepatic, Hormone Precursors, Infusion, Laxative, Lotion, Nervine, Parasiticide, Pectoral, Sedative, Stimulants, Tincture, Tonics, Urinary Antiseptic, Vasodilator.

Herbs For Females

Some Useful Formulas

Common Herbal Formulas in Chemists and Health Shops

Herbal

Aniseed, Angelica, Black Cohosh, Blue Cohosh, Beth Root, Black Haw, Chamomile, Dandelion, Cramp Bark, Damiana, Dong Quai, False Unicorn Root, Feverfew, Fenugreek, Ginseng (Panax), Ginseng (Siberian), Ginger, Hops Hops, Ladys Mantle, Maca,Milk Thistle, Motherwort, Passion Flower, Raspberry, Red Clover, Rosemary, Sage, St Johns Wort, Schizandra, Sarsaparilla, Shepherds Purse, Skullcap, Squaw Vine, Valerian, Vervain, Vitex (Chaste Tree), Yarrow, Wild Yam, Withania, Zizyphus.

Introduction

I wrote this over a decade ago but now here the laws have changed and I am not allowed to prescribe without seeing the patient so I have had to change this from being a Kit with medicine supplied to just giving you the recipe of the remedies used in the Kit. The Kit was designed originally for people in remote areas in outback Australia where there can be little help for the day to day problems and specialists only pop up every six months if you are lucky. It was designed to empower the patient and give simple and safe treatment using Homoeopathic Remedies whose formula I kept secret but will now give to the world. I have always been upset by the way our modern medical system seeks to disempower you and leave you stranded and dependent on them. A good example I have helped many women with and you can now do so yourself is where some poor women in the middle of the desert finds a lump in her breast, a mammogram machine is hundreds of miles away, the fuel costs are high, money is tight. Now there is stress and worry on top of all the other burdens. This book will tell you to wait till the darkest of night and then put a torch under the breast (Translumination) which allows you to see through the breast. Looking down at the breast if you see a lump that the light can still penetrate means that the lump is liquid filled and may be a fluid filled cyst. If you see the lump and no light passes through then it is a solid mass and may be a tumor so you have to get medical help immediately. I have rewritten most of this book and added my latest experiences especially in the cancer part and added a Homoeopathic Section where I give you the formula for the medicines used in the original kit. I will now let you read the old Foreword and original add for the kit.

Regards

Mark Gilberd

Old Foreword

This booklet and kit has been designed and made for practical people who are not afraid to take their own fate in their hands and do something about it. The booklet is set out in such a way as to empower you and put the control of your health back into your hands where it belongs. To many people in this life just sit back and do little to improve their health while the reality is that if you have been on a junk food diet all your life and spend 30 hours or more in front of the TV a week your chances of getting healthy again regardless how much medication you take are very slim.

This booklet gives you information about Menopause and introduces you to the common symptoms and gives you a way of recording your own personal symptoms in a way that will show up any type of pattern that might be happening. Latter we go into diet and show how this can affect some of the symptoms and health in general and then we move on to supplements that can be taken which work to increase your health and relieve your symptoms. After the supplements we move to a section that gives you most of the products you will find in Health Shops and Chemists that are used for Menopause and we list the ingredients of each so you can look up the individual herbs in the Herbal and see if they match your Symptoms. We also give you some common Herbal Formulas that have been used over time.

Now we move onto a Herbal which contains about 40 of the main female Herbs and has a write up about each along with their Actions (A herbal actions list follows the Herbal) on the body. Not only can we use this section for reference but we can also use it to formulate our own personal formulas matching our personal symptoms.

Over the page we show you how to use the Homoeopathic Complexes which are the medications supplied with the booklet that you yourself can mix in such a way as to cover your own personal symptoms.

If after this you are still having problems then you could move onto Herbal treatment which can be very effective but the most important thing is that by then you would of done most of the ground work yourself. For example your nutrition would of improved, you would also be taking the correct nutritional supplements for your condition, you would have your own symptom chart which would probably be showing a pattern by now so you would of covered a lot of ground and be well on the way to a healthier future.

Last of all I want to say especially to people with severe problems don't be afraid of using Hormone Treatment that Doctors usually prescribe for severe problems as this form of treatment can bring reasonably fast relief and you can use this treatment to get yourself over the worst of the problems then slowly wean yourself off as your health improves. Problems with hormone replacement therapy seem only to happen to the long time users but if you use it just to get yourself over the worst and improve your health while you are doing this and keep on using your chart you should come out alright at the end.

Well best of luck

Mark Gilberd
Homoeopath   Medical Herbalist
Iridologist

Registered with the Australian Traditional Society in each Modality

Menopause Kit

This is a unique product designed for women who live in remote areas and who have to travel great distances to see a Doctor. It gives all the information you need on how to treat the problem symptoms and a system of recording your own personal symptoms (Symptom Diary) which will help to show you the future problems you may expect and is a valuable record for a Doctors future reference as it shows the Doctor patterns and obliges them to act.. The Kit contains a Booklet giving you the information you need with sections on Causes, The Common Symptoms of Menopause, Symptoms In Detail with Supplements and Herb Lists, Diet and Nutrition, Common Supplements, Common Menopause Formulas in The Chemists and Health Shops (with ingredients listed so you can look them up in the Herbal) and at the back of the booklet there is a Comprehensive Herbal with 40 Female suitable herbs, a list of 38 different Herbal Actions along with the Herbs and lots more. The last page is devoted to the use of the Homoeopathic Complexes that are a part of the kit and it teaches you how to use them to match your personal symptoms.

The Kit comes with 4 Homoeopathic Complexes.

There are 4 Stock Bottles in the kit and they are labeled

Meno A : Which is the main remedy to which the others are added.(Contains Homoeopathic Estrogen)

Meno B : Add to A for the relief of **Depression, Emotions, Mood Changes and Headaches**.

Meno C : Add to A for the relief of **Pains and Cramps**.

Meno D : Add to A for the relief of **Vaginal Pain, Dryness and Incontinence**.

<u>Meno A :</u> is the main remedy, for this remedy has the hormone Estrogen in it. The other remedies can be added to your dose to counter other symptoms as and when they occur.

The Kit also has a separate Acid and Alkaline Chart and Nutrition Guide.

This chart allows you to see if your body may be excessively acid. If this is the case your body may be stealing minerals from your bones or anywhere it can to make the body more alkaline especially the blood and in turn this could lead to osteoporosis. Excessively acid bodies may lead to arthritis and other diseases. The nutrition section includes Nutrition For The Reproductive System and an introduction to the herb Maca which slowly over time may rejuvenate the endocrine system.

Feel better and take control of your life today.

The Menopause Time Line
Perimenopause
2 to 8 years before the last menstrual period and 1 year after

1. Decreased fertility
2. Irregular Periods
3. Increased PMS
4. Heavy bleeding may occur within periods.
5. Sex drive my decrease due to a drop in Testosterone
6. Decreased estrogen levels
7. Hot flushes and night sweats may begin.

You may experience a few or many of these symptoms

Headaches, fibroid tumors, breast pain and lumps, fatigue, anxiety, emotional volatility, hot flushes, foggy thinking, depression, hair loss, unwanted facial hair, weight gain and night sweats.

Some of these symptoms may continue into menopause

Menopause

1. Ovulation ceases
2. Thinning and drying of mucous membranes of vagina and urethra
3. Hot flushes and night sweats
4. Insomnia

Post Menopause

1. Skin becomes thin
2. Cholesterol levels increase
3. Bones become more brittle, increased risk of fractures, osteoporosis may happen
4. Muscle tone loss
5. Increased risk of heart disease and cancer
6. Hot flushes may continue

Lots of these can be prevented that's what the book is all about

Taking The Fear Out Of Menopause

Before we get into finding out what menopause really is lets destroy some of the myths associated with it and get back to good old common sense after all menopause has been happening since the human race has been around so what's all the fuss now.

We hear a lot about the emotional problems that come along with menopause but is this really all the menopauses fault. Menopause usually happens somewhere from the ages of 45 to 55. In this period of our lives lots of things are happening and lots of new decisions have to be made, for example - between these ages most of our kids have grown up and will be leaving home, for some this will be a time of sadness and no doubt others will be dancing around the house but it also leads to other problems such as do we really want to keep this big house, do I really want to stay with my partner now the kids are gone, and for some of us when the kids leave then our own parents seem to start going downhill and start to need a lot of help and care.

So the reality is at the time of menopause there are usually a lot more things happening in your life then there normally are and a lot of these things are very emotional situations which would be very emotional situations if they happened at any other time of your life anyway.

So what can we do? The answer to this is to be prepared and the way we are going to do this is to make our own Personal Plan. We shall start by gathering intelligence about the enemy especially about what the enemy does and how it acts and then we shall see just where exactly the enemy positions are at the moment so we know what to expect. After we know what's happening then it's time for us to plan our attack and if all goes well we will not just make it through the menopause but into a long and healthy life with not to many problems.

Before we get to far ahead one important thing must be mentioned that is always over looked and that is people who are healthy and haven't really had any health problems through their lives seem to sail through menopause without any serious problems while those who aren't in the best of health and have had lots of problems through their lives are the ones that seem to have the most problems at menopause so if you are not healthy now's the time to get healthy.

So what's the exact meaning of Menopause anyway - Menopause means the final menstruation and comes from Greek meaning month and cessation. Perimenopause is Greek for around or near menopause and refers to the time of change.

The real word we should be using is The Climacteric which is an old Greek word meaning "a step in the ladder". The Climacteric means all the changes that happen from the first symptoms of change to the final symptoms of menopause. (This is a word that you will come across in medical writings but for this booklet we shall just use the term menopause). A women of 50 plus is estimated to be infertile after a period of 12 months from her last menstruation

As mentioned before the common ages for menopause are 45 to 55, listed below are some percentage figures from statistics of the onset of menopause.

1/. By the age of 47 the onset of menopause is about 25%

2/. By the age of 50 the onset of menopause is about 50%

3/. By the age of 52 the onset of menopause is about 75%

4/.By the age of 55 the onset of menopause is about 100%

Now that we have a idea of when to expect it lets move on to how the change happens and what causes it.

What Happens And The Cause

The actual cause of the beginning of menopause is that the ovaries are getting close to their use by date and are failing to respond to the actions of the hormones that are trying to stimulate them to produce more eggs. When this happens the body responds by increasing the production of stimulating hormones and so begins all the hormone imbalances. Before menopause, changes in the hormone balance have been going on for some time. Symptoms may have been noticed for anything up to ten years before the periods stop. Often menstruation does not end suddenly but becomes irregular with periods coming less frequently although in some they can come more frequently. Sometimes for some women the bleeding can become less and less with each period and other women can have flooding. If flooding becomes regular it is best to have a checkup as flooding is one of the main symptoms of fibroids which are fairly common at the menopause age.

As menopause approaches the relationship between the pituitary gland and the ovaries is upset with FSH (Follicle Stimulating Hormone) and LH (Luteinizing Hormone) levels going much higher as the body tries to stimulate the poor tired ovaries to produce more. This process can be described as rather nastily but accurately as "trying to flog a dead horse" and leads to large quantities of the mentioned hormones and low quantities of estrogen and progesterone the hormones they are trying to force the poor ovaries to produce.

As the ovaries decrease production and the cycles change a type of estrogen is produced by the adrenal glands which can replace up to 75% of the premenopausal levels in some women right up until their seventies. Other women, due to poor health unfortunately produce much less. Estrogen is also produced in small amounts from body fat so thin women run the risk of producing less. Another source of estrogen can be the conversion of androgen the male hormone made also in the adrenal glands into estrogen by the liver and fat tissues.

All of this replacement estrogen is the body's natural efforts to minimize the transition of the menopause and to try to make it as problem free as possible.

After reading the above you can see how some very healthy women manage to get through menopause without too much trouble for if you are in good shape and not under stress your healthy adrenal glands should be able to work at maximum output producing estrogen and your healthy liver should be able to convert androgens to estrogen with out to much effort along with a little help from the fat cells. Let's now look at a woman whose health is not too good. Due to the adrenal glands being not as good as they should the glands output of estrogen is much lower, remember what we mentioned before about life's problems all coming at once - the kids leaving etc. all this stress reduces the adrenal glands out put more (especially if you are an emotional person) along with a poor diet and hypoglycemia etc. and if the liver is not working so good either as it isn't in most people with our modern diet and pollution the output of estrogen is further reduced leaving you wide open to all the problems of menopause.

So the most important point is Get Healthy Now.

What Are Hormones

The word hormone comes from the Greek word horman, which means to stir up, or arouse to activity. This is a good description for it is exactly what hormones do. Hormones are made in small glands throughout the body and from there use the blood circulation to travel to their destination. Each one has a specific job to do on its target organ or tissue, usually controlling, activating or directing certain functions. Many hormones can have an effect on your urges, desires, feelings and emotions just by the different strengths and mixtures that they are working at. Fluctuating hormone levels will vary throughout your life but there main fluctuating moments will be in Adolescence and Menopause which you could say is the reverse of Adolescence.

Hormones when you are young trigger your growth spurts especially at puberty, then throughout your life they control the speed of your metabolism at one extreme maybe making you a skinny high speed workaholic while at the other extreme a slow individual who is prone to putting on weight. Hormones balance your blood sugar and also have an effect on your bodies water balance along with affecting your breathing and the nervous system. To a certain degree hormones rule so we have to be very careful before we start playing around with this complex system.

As mentioned before some women can live their whole life and have no problems with this system while others have known nothing but problems. Hormonal upsets can arise from the use of the birth control pill or other hormone containing medicines or more natural conditions such as pregnancy or from a miscarriage. Surgery and operations such as hysterectomy or sterilization or even violence and mental trauma can throw the hormone system out of whack and lead on to many unwanted and annoying symptoms. Stress, lifestyle and genetic inheritance are major factors in hormone problems with each needing an investigation if problems are arising, sometimes it can be as simple as just changing your lifestyle while at other times it may be disease related such as the onset of Adult Diabetes.

Let's have a look at the three main hormones affected by menopause.

Estrogen

Estrogen is not really a single hormone but a class of

hormones that control things such as growth, the function of the female sex organs, secondary sexual characteristics, Calcium absorption etc. Estrogen includes hormones such as estradiol and estrone which are essential for the health of the reproductive organs, and estriol which is the predominant estrogen hormone during pregnancy. Estradiol is the main estrogen. Prior to menopause it is the dominant form of estrogen in the body. Estrone is an inactive or weak form of estrogen which the body produces after menopause in the fat tissues.

As a fetus your body began producing estrogen when you were 15 to 20 weeks old, at puberty your levels of estrogen increased dramatically and maybe even erratically and from then on your life became influenced by the cyclic monthly changes. Then along comes menopause which is kind of the reverse of adolescence.

Progesterone

Progesterone is produced mainly by the ovaries, with a small amount produced by the adrenal glands. During pregnancy the placenta produces large amounts. Progesterone is also needed for the production of other hormones such as cortisol which plays an important role in the metabolism of carbohydrates, fats and proteins and in the body's response to injury and infection. The production of ovarian progesterone declines during the menopausal years.

Follicle Stimulating Hormone (FSH) -

Produced by the pituitary gland to stimulate the ovaries to get follicles growing. This is the hormone that starts the menstrual cycle.

Luteinising Hormone (LH) - Produced by the pituitary gland to get the follicle to release the egg.

Testosterone

As well as being the main hormone for men testosterone is also important to women. Half of a women's testosterone is produced in the ovaries and the other half in the adrenal glands. Testosterone helps to determine secondary sexual chrematistics such as muscle mass, patterns of hair growth and sexual desire. Testosterone levels reduce about one third in the average post-menopausal women, if the ovaries are removed the fall is twice as great.

Conclusion

With so many hormones in the body each doing their own thing but at the same time influencing many other hormones, sometimes the best way to go is to try to balance the lot of them instead of picking on individuals. This can be a great benefit especially to people prone to other problems such as Adult Onset Diabetes. The best herb to do this is Maca. This herb is known as an Adaptogen, which means it tries to adapt the body to get the best you can out of it under the present conditions. It is a good herb for the transition especially if you have a lot of stress in your life. I prefer using this herb in powder form and I think it also works out cheaper this way.

Maca

Actions - Nutritive, increases energy and stamina, adaptogen, helps to restore the endocrine system eg ovaries, pancreas, thyroid, adrenals etc.

Maca is a root vegetable only grown in Peru, indigenous to the Andean Mountains. It is a turnip like tuber that has a pleasant malty butterscotch like flavor and has been used for well over 5000 years. Like other herbs grown at high altitudes in extreme weather conditions (eg - Ginseng) this herbs packs quiet a punch especially nutrition wise.

Maca strengthens and balances the endocrine system and has a positive effect on the organs which become more balanced and stronger. Areas Maca may help in are PMS, Menopause, Hot Flushes, Frigidity, Chronic Fatigue, Anemia, Infertility, Breast Feeding and much more. Some people even use it as a HRT replacement.

When shopping for Maca remember that it only comes from the Peruvian highlands and only the root of the plant is used

This little write up is only an introduction to you of Maca and how it may benefit you, I will leave it to you to do your own research. I have been using Maca on patients for years now and only really started using it for its nutrition and energy giving properties and always kind of used it as a background remedy. Now I really pay attention to it as an endocrine balancer especially to the adrenal glands. Now it's your turn to see what it can do. Being a Adaptogen this is a long term use herb give it at least 6 months so it can supply the nutrition and fine tune the body. Adaptogens adapt your body to suit you and your circumstances and this cannot be done overnight.

Other Adaptogens in the Herbal - Withania, Ginseng, Siberian Ginseng and Schizandra.

Warning - Maca is very rich in nutrients so start with small doses like a quarter of a teaspoon and slowly over a few weeks build up to the recommended dose.

Pharmaceutical HRT Questionnaire

This is an example of a questionnaire that Pharmaceutical Companies give out to determine if women with menopausal symptoms are in need of Hormone Replacement Therapy. They advise that if you score above 15 you probably need HRT. Some people put this to test and found young male athletes got the highest scores followed by mothers with young children and then menopause aged women. The chart is here for your interest and use. I would only be worried if I got a very high score. Remember all the information in this book is to allow you to help yourself especially if you live in remote areas. You may wish to fill it out so you can show your remote area traveling specialist so they are forced to do something about it now instead of six months' time when they come back.

HRT Questionnaire

Rate each of the following problems with zero as no problem, one as mild, two as moderate and three as severe. Then total up your score.

Lightheadedness

Headaches

Irritability

Depression

Feelings Of Being Unloved

Anxiety
Mood changes
Hot Flushes
Sleeplessness
Unusual Fatigue
Backache
Joint Pains
Muscle Pains
Increased Facial Hair
Crawling Feelings Under The Skin
Decreased Libido
Dry Skin Or Genitals
Dry Skin Arms Legs And Body
Uncomfortable Intercourse
Urinary Frequency

Total Score

Common Symptoms Of Menopause

According to surveys in Britain 16 to 30% of all menopausal women experience no uncomfortable symptoms at all and of the 70% that do only 10% of them consider their symptoms bad enough to have treatment. Interestingly enough there are far more than the 10% receiving Hormone Replacement Treatment but this is not surprising considering the drug companies interest in profit. I will now give a short list of the most common symptoms but won't go into any detail with them as we are going to do this latter, the most common symptoms are -

1. Hot flashes or flushes
2. Night sweats
3. Vaginal dryness and itching
4. Thinning of the vaginal tissue - painful sex
5. Osteoporosis - bone pains
6. Mood swings and depression - emotions
7. Fuzzy thinking - forgetfulness -confusion
8. Sleep problems
9. Headaches
10. Palpitations, breathlessness.

There are lots more symptoms then this, but these are the fairly common ones. Now that we have got to know menopause a bit better it's time to see how it is effecting us and find out where we are up to in the path that the menopause takes. To do this we are going to start to make our own personal chart. This chart will be about a yearlong and is actually a diary which is going to show your periods and your symptoms.

Menstrual Diary Chart

Day	January	February	March	April
1	B	HBD	M	
2	B	MP	M	
3	BHBD	MP	M	
4	HBD	M		
5	HBD	M		
6	MP	M		
7	MP			
8	M			
9	M			
10	M			
11				
12				D
13				BD
14				BD
15				BD
16				BD
18				HBD
19			D	MP
20			BD	M
21			BDHBD	M
22		D	HBD	M
23		BD	MP	M
24		HBD	MP	
25		HBD	M	
26	B	HBD	M	
27	B	MP	M	
28	BD	M		
29	HBD			
30	HBD			

Making Your Own Chart

Above is an example chart. Jane is using this chart to plot her PMS symptoms and on her chart she will be looking for the same things that we will be looking for and they are patterns. Examples are, are my period patterns changing, are the symptoms getting worse or better, are the symptoms following a pattern, are they coming in groups etc.

Keeping this record is a must, especially if you live in a remote area as this is what the book was originally designed for. Generally specialists get into remote areas once every six months if you are lucky and as these charts are a main diagnostic tool you need to have one ready or you may be asked to fill one out and have to wait another six months for treatment. If you are armed with this chart before you see a Doctor or a specialist you should expect good and accurate treatment, if you are not happy go to another Doctor and get a second opinion. As mentioned before people who have had very little trouble through their lives will generally not have much trouble with menopause but those of you who have had PMS problems or other hormonal problem may well have a more difficult time so it is best to be armed with all the information you can.

Keeping this record puts you in control of your life for you know what's happening to you and what has happened to you in the past and to a certain extent you should be able to predict what could happen in the future especially if you start seeing patterns. Now that you know what is happening to you treatment for the symptoms can be sort and as you keep on plotting your chart you will be able to tell if this treatment is helping you, for if it is the symptoms on the chart should be receding and if they are staying the same or getting worse then you know this treatment is not for you and you can try something else.

There is a code that is used on the chart, if you can't see your symptoms there then add your own, don't forget this as it is very important. Every time a symptom comes along use the code and put it on the chart.

Code to The Chart

M = Menstrual Bleeding

D = Depression

H = Headache

B = Breast pain

P = Period pain

F = Hot Flushes

Do not be afraid to add your own symptoms to the chart as the larger the picture the better. It is the pattern of the symptoms you see in the future that will tell you if the symptoms are hormonally related.

Symptoms In Detail

We will now go into detail about the common symptoms of menopause and mention some of the nutritional supplements which may help to relieve the symptoms as well as some herbs. With Herbal treatment it is best to get this done professionally making sure of course that you bring along your chart with you. The reason for this is that an herbalist will treat you holistically and not just the most bothersome symptoms also they know about the interactions with any medicine you may be taking. This is very important and the best way to show you is to give you an example of how I might treat someone with menopause problems.

Usually when I make a Herbal prescription which is usually in tincture form I try to use no more than 5 herbs and for a women with menopause problems one herb would go to help the liver which now has the extra job of converting androgen to estrogen, another herb might go to help the adrenal glands which are now doing the main job of making estrogen especially in a person who is under a lot of stress physically or mentally and my remaining herbs would go to helping the main symptoms of the case but with these I would try to choose herbs that could be converted into hormones easily. So as you can now see there is a lot more that goes into it then just prescribing herbs for the symptoms. When you come to the Herbal Section we will give you a lot more information in Herbs Used For Females.

Hot Flashes, Flushes and Night Sweats

Depending on which surveys you look at the figures for women who experience flushes vary but are around about 60 to 75%. Unfortunately what is not shown is the severity of the symptoms which are variable. The flushes may be very quick in which case they are called flashes while the longer ones are known as flushes; typically they occur several times a day and last a few minutes at a time. Some women report them occurring several times a week for up to a year while others at worst say several times a day for 5 years. The worst flushes can have with them palpitations, dizziness or faintness and can be very frightening.

Hot flushes usually begin when the periods are still regular or are just starting to fluctuate and are often the first indications that menopause is approaching. The cause is not really known (estrogen withdrawal symptoms?) but it obviously involves the nervous systems action on the capillaries which cause vasomotor changes which lead to sudden hot sensations and flushing, especially of the face and neck often followed by a chill or perspiration as the heat fades. Hot weather, emotional stress, exercise, alcohol and certain foods (spices) can make the symptoms worse or bring them on. A helpful suggestion is to dress in layers so as you heat up you can remove a layer at a time etc. Night sweats are probably related and would share the same cause. An example of night sweats at their worst would be a women throwing off her blankets after soaking the sheets with sweat and then feeling cold a few minutes later and having to put the blankets back on. This can go on for a few months or a few years.

I think diet has a lot to do with the problem, Japanese women don't seem to be very effected by flushes and there diet is high in essential fatty acids from fish while our diet is not. Some people now think that hypoglycemia (low blood sugar) may be a cause so this is worth getting checked. Consider baking the Linda Kearns Hormone Cake which is given later on in the book and see what happens. Stress also plays a major part as well so try to remove some of your stressors or try some sort of meditation or another form of relaxation. Deep breathing exercises have given good results. If you are keeping a Symptoms Dairy make sure you mark down the hot flushes as they sometimes follow a pattern which you may be able to figure out.

Exercise - Regular and moderate exercise may decrease FSH and LH levels, reducing and even eliminating symptoms. Exercise can often restore or help to stabilize hormone levels. Exercise also exercises the capillaries and should tone them up which should also relieve symptoms. Add to this Hesperidin and you should hopefully have good results.

Nutritional Treatment

1/. Vitamin E in the form of d alpha-tocopherol 300 IU twice per day has helped some women with hot flushes. In the 1940s women with cancer or prone to cancer were given vitamin E with good results that were well documented because they couldn't get estrogen because of their cancer risk. Vitamin E is a hormone normalizer. Tests have shown that when E is low the levels of FSH and LH increase. As these levels are high anyway in women going through menopause a lack of E could make the problem far worse. Cutting down or eliminating sugar, caffeine, alcohol and hot spicy food can help this condition. Other symptoms that are helped by vitamin E are nervousness, fatigue, insomnia, dizziness, heart palpations, shortness of breath and vaginal dryness.

Caution - No one taking anticoagulant drugs for thrombosis or other similar conditions should take Vitamin E.

2/. Evening Primrose Oil or **Borage Oil** (starflower oil) have a reputation for relieving hot flushes in high doses, take up to 1000 mg two or three times a day or **EPA** from fish oils. A good multi vitamin and mineral pill may be of benefit especially if the diet is poor.

3/. Tryptophan 500mg (Amino Acid) - Can help with flushes and night sweats. See supplement section.

4/. Hesperidin or Bioflavonoids - Bioflavonoids have been used successfully to reduce hot flashes as well as to reduce heavy bleeding. They also help protect and strengthen capillary walls. This helps to reduce hot flashes by improving the walls of the capillaries venous tone, restoring normal capillary permeability and improving lymphatic drainage. Take 500mgs 3 times daily with 500mgs of Vitamin C as long as you have symptoms. The main bioflavonoids are rutin, quercetin, citrin, hesperidin, genestein and diadzein.

Herbal Treatment

Herbs used to treat flushing and sweating are usually based on estrogen and progesterone promoting herbs. The best ones are Maca, Sage , Black Cohosh, Dong Quai and Vitex. Other are Wild Yam, Red Clover, Lady's Mantle, Motherwort, Siberian Ginseng and Schizandra.

A infusion of Sage is effective if sipped throughout the day. (keep in the fridge).

Vitex Agnus Castus - Is regarded throughout Europe as the herb for menopause and PMS. It stimulates the pituitary (hormone control center) function altering FSH and LH secretions. Used for 3 months it will increase your levels of natural progesterone and help control hot flushes, depression and a dry vagina. Caution do not use with the birth control pill.

Zizyphus - This is the new kid on the block that is being used in a lot of the new menopause formulas and also sleeping remedies. This herb has been used in Chinese medicine for over 4000 years. One write up

I read said, The seed is used in TCM to quieten the spirit, for dream disturbed sleep, insomnia, irritability, palpations with anxiety and spontaneous night sweats.

Look up individual herbs in the herbal to see if they suit your symptoms.

Anxiety, Depression, Mood Swings and Emotions

Anxiety and mood swings are very upsetting for some menopausal women and may continue for some time, possibly alternating with feelings of depression. Irritability and weepiness are common and may be greeted unsympathetically by some family members. Moods may lift as quickly as they come and the sea saw pattern of these emotions can be difficult to handle (make sure you are putting them on the chart). It helps to bear in mind that this is just a passing phase.

Symptoms of hormonally related depression are insomnia, early morning waking, poor appetite and sometimes loss of weight and if you suffered from depression before menopause your chances of suffering depression at menopause are far greater. Depression is often a physical as well as a psychological problem reflected in poor energy levels so it might be wise to treat the energy levels before the depression. If you had PMS problems before menopause it is not uncommon for a lot of these problems to continue into menopause.

The problem here with this group of symptoms is that so many things can be happening at once not only with hormone levels all over the place but with your social life all over the place especially with the problems we were talking about at the beginning of the book with maybe the kids leaving home, parents getting sick etc. Maybe it's time to go for a nice long holiday.

Nutritional Treatment

Stimulants can cause sudden changes in the moods and emotions especially caffeine and alcohol.

If you suffer from depression scrutinize your diet to make sure your blood sugar levels remain as constant as possible. If you have a problem stabilizing your blood sugar you may want to supplement chromium or try the herb Fenugreek. The Bs and Magnesium are the ones to try first as they may give you a yes or no answer to your problems very quickly.

1/. Chromium - Helps to improve efficient use of insulin and keeps blood sugar levels steady Take 100 to 200 micrograms once or twice a day.

2/. Tryptophan 500mg (Amino Acid) - Can help with some types of depression. See supplement section.

3/.Glutamine (Amino Acid) - Helps to improve mental clarity, fatigue, reduces blood sugar, reduces sugar cravings, alleviates aggressiveness, improves mood, improves concentration and lifts depression. Take 500 to 1000mg twice daily for 3 months.

4/. B6 is very effective, B12 and B Complex -
See supplement section. For anxiety it would be better
to take the complex as all the bs tend to work
together. Get a pack where they are all about 50mg,
have one in the morning and one before you go to
sleep that way its trapped in the body till the
morning.

5/. Magnesium is the most important mineral to
take for this condition. The nervous system runs on
Calcium and Magnesium so make sure there is plenty
there.

Herbal Treatment

Skullcap, Valerian, Chamomile, Rosemary, Damiana,
St Johns Wort, Vervain, Motherwort, Zizyphus.

Have a look at Maca if you have constant fatigue.
Most of these herbs are nervines, try a cup of
chamomile tea especially for anxiety as it is best to
keep it simple.

See **Anti-depressive Herbs** in the Herbal Actions List

Foggy Thinking

Having trouble remembering conversations or recent
events, do you keep on losing your keys, are you
having difficulty at work remembering what you
need too. Sometimes declining levels of both
estrogens and progesterone can lead to foggy
thinking. There can be lots of other reasons such as
regular drinking depleting all the B vitamins needed
by the brain, lack of zinc, not enough sugar as the

brain requires lots of energy to function properly, another possibility is a poor blood supply to the head. Another problem can be lack of the essential fatty acids because our brain and spinal cords are mostly made of fat and need it to regenerate. Exercise can be a great help by improving you blood circulation.

Nutritional Treatment

B Vits - Try in a medium dose complex (50mg) for a week and you should get a yes or no answer fairly fast.

Iron - The brain needs lots of oxygen to function well, with iron being the main oxygen carrier a shortage can slow down thinking.

Herbal Treatment

Ginkgo Biloba

This herb opens up the arteries going to the head and allows a better blood flow, which in turn brings in more oxygen and glucose which are the main needs of the brain. This herb combines well with the herbs below and I use it generally with any herb that I want to push into the head.

Brahmi

Brahmi has been used in traditional Indian medicine for over 3000 years. It has been used to treat conditions such as fluid retention, chronic skin conditions, high cholesterol levels, epileptic fits, depression including post natal depression, frigidity, irregular menstruation, mental and physical fatigue, exhaustion, restlessness, insomnia and over active mind, mental deterioration of the elderly, forgetfulness, confused and cloudy thoughts, anxiety, ADD, stress, hysteria, nervous breakdown, insanity and to improve circulation. Brahmi is valued as a nerve and brain tonic and widely used by students for improving mental clarity, confidence, intelligence, concentration and memory recall. Brahmi as herbal supplements and tablets have been marketed for super learning, for memory and as a brain tonic.

Schizandra

This herb is mainly focused on the liver and is used for under function and damage to this organ. Schizandra improves mental, physical and sensory performance and helps in the handling of stress and increases stamina. This herb can also help with night sweats and improve a poor memory and is good for the treatment of depression.

Tiredness And Fatigue

If this is caused from insomnia read that section. Like a lot of problems associated with menopause they don't really know the cause of this problem and some would not even relate it to menopause. One thing to check if this gets really bad is the thyroid as a under active thyroid makes you feel tired, lets you put on weight very easily and can have other symptoms of constipation, dry skin and maybe depression. Two more areas to check are your iron levels as you may becoming anemic especially if you have been having heavy bleeding and the other area is hypoglycemia you could have low blood sugar. If you are still having problems and can't find a solution cut sugar out of the diet and focus on a good diet based on complex carbohydrates. Then start a course of Maca for 3 months. Maca will balance the hormones and supply nutrition and its adaptogen action will help with the fatigue. Adaptogens do just what the name implies; they make you adapt to get the best you can possibly get out of yourself. These are the herbs we use for chronic fatigue, AIDS and Cancer. Other examples are Astragalus and Withania.

Nutritional Treatment

Make sure your diet is good and has plenty of complex carbohydrates in it, take a natural iron supplement if needed, the seaweeds and kelp are good foods for the thyroid.

Magnesium - This mineral is often deficient in women who consume a diet that is high in refined carbohydrates and sugar. **Such diets deplete the body of the minerals chromium, manganese, zinc, magnesium and the B complex vitamins.** Women with magnesium deficiency often crave sugar and in particular chocolate.

Food sources - lettuce, garlic, tomatoes, potatoes, raisins, bananas, almonds, cashews, dates, most whole grains, wheat germ, spinach, peas, celery.

Tryptophan (Amino Acid) - Low levels of this are associated with anxiety and insomnia in menopausal women. See supplement section.

Glutamine (Amino Acid) - Helps to improve

mental clarity, fatigue, reduces blood sugar, reduces sugar cravings, alleviates aggressiveness, improves mood, improves concentration and lifts depression. Take 500 to 1000mg twice daily for 3 months.

Herbal Treatment

Be careful here as most of the herbs that people would prescribe would probably be stimulants which in the long run would make you worse, try getting energy from your diet first and if this is not successful think of the Adaptogen herbs like Siberian Ginseng and Withania.

Look up individual herbs in the herbal to see if they suit your symptoms.

Insomnia

The many hormonal changes that occur when you are approaching menopause can disturb a previously sound sleeper. One of the best thing you can do is try to go to sleep and wake up at the same time each day, forcing the body into a pattern. If you are not on Maca or the Hormone Cake try the simple specifics for insomnia. Sometimes a deficiency in Magnesium can cause you to wake up repeatedly during the night or suffer from frequent sleeplessness. This condition effects everyone now and again and it is best to try the simple remedies to get over this such as hot milk etc. Avoid caffeine in any drinks especially close to bed time. Concentrate on the herbs below.

Nutritional Treatment

Vitamin B12 - Many studies have found that B12 promotes sleep, especially in people with sleep disorders. As yet they do not know why but it could be an idea to try and get a fast yes or no answer.

Tryptophan (Amino Acid) - Low levels of this are associated with anxiety and insomnia in menopausal women. See supplement section.

Magnesium, especially if you have a lot of stress in your life.

Herbal Treatment

Chamomile tea is effective and is what I use, other herbs which can be used alone or mixed together to improve the wanted action are Passion Flower, Lemon Balm, Skullcap, Valerian and Hops, Zizyphus.

Hops would be a good long term herb to think of because it helps make estrogen and also has a good action on the digestive system. Now you know where the term brewers droop comes from. When beer replaced mead and became a major crop, lots of women who were going through menopause while they were harvesting the hops noticed an improvement in their condition, this is due to the sap working like an essential oil on the skin and medicating the blood stream.

Look up individual herbs in the herbal to see if they suit your symptoms.

Headaches

Hormonal headaches in perimenopausal women usually occur before, during and sometimes after the period. If you had these headaches before menopause then you are most likely to have them through the menopause. This is where the chart comes in handy as every time you have a headache chart it and if after a time we can see a pattern then we know that the hormones are responsible and it's not a migraine or something else. If the headaches are hormonal they usually come on after a big slump in the estrogen levels and may be associated with general body aches and pains, fatigue and depression. I think here we should plan our attack at the beginning because once the headache seems to get settled it is very hard to get rid of so as soon as you feel the first symptoms coming on take the main remedy in the kit for this has estrogen in it.

Check your blood sugar levels as well especially if you are a chocolate craver at these times. I will only give a few treatment listings for this because it should really be treated holistically with the other symptoms. I will mention this though, lots of women who have had regular bad headaches for years and years and have been taking pain killers for them have actually been having hormone headaches that could of been cured with estrogen, unfortunately years of painkillers have now damaged their kidneys.

Nutritional Treatment

Evening Primrose Oil is an effective treatment for

headaches.

Herbal Treatment

Feverfew is a good preventative for migraines and Withania can help with severe pain.

Effective herbs for headaches are Chamomile, Feverfew, Hops, Peppermint, Rosemary, St Johns Wort, Skullcap, Valerian and Withania. Wood Betony is used for painful facial pains.

Look up individual herbs in the herbal to see if they suit your symptoms.

Fluid Retention or Oedema (bloating)

The symptoms here are similar to the ones that women with PMS get which are swelling of the hands and feet, facial area, abdomen and pelvic area. The fluid retention can be of certain areas or everywhere. This can also account for a large weight gain. The cause of this is the hormone aldosterone (regulates fluids) being upset by the fluctuations in the other hormones.

Nutritional Treatment

Avoid salt as salt holds water in the body, vitamin and mineral supplements that may help include magnesium, Vitamin E, Evening Primrose Oil and **Vitamin B6**. An organic wholefood diet with plenty of unrefined carbohydrates will help, as this removes toxic byproducts from the tissues that are retaining the fluid. Massage may also help in this case but only a short gentle one as you may overload the system with toxins that the water filled cells were holding.

Herbal Treatment

Dandelion leaf infusion is the best way to go here as it is the best diuretic because it puts more potassium into the body then it takes out (all diuretic take out potassium) and is fairly gentle to the system. Have a look at the Diuretic list in the Herbal Actions Section.

Dysmenorrhea And Flooding

Dysmenorrhea simply means painful menstruation and there are two different types one being Spasmodic Dysmenorrhea which is the cramp like pains and the other Congestive Dysmenorrhea where pain starts well before the period and is often due to inflammatory problems with the uterus such as endometriosis, fibroids, pelvic inflammatory disease or problems with the ovary such as ovarian cysts. Pain is due to congestion in the pelvic area. It usually occurs latter in reproductive life after the age of 30 or after childbirth. The major symptoms are feelings of aching heaviness in the lower abdomen and legs, the thighs may be especially painful. Accompanying diarrhea is not uncommon. The discomfort is usually relieved once bleeding starts.

Irregular Periods And Flooding - Fluctuating hormone levels can interrupt the ovulation cycle causing you to ovulate on some months and not on others. If you do not ovulate you don't produce enough progesterone to have a period so the lining of your uterus builds up so next time when everything works as normal you have more lining to shed causing flooding.

Herbal Treatment

Antispasmodic and analgesic herbs can provide relief to symptoms of pains with cramps but longer term treatment would include uterine toners and hormone balancers. With the congestive form you really have to find the cause. For the irregular periods and flooding along with the above symptoms look at the herbs below.

Beth Root

Actions - Uterine tonic, astringent, expectorant, antispasmodic alterative.

Contains natural precursors of the female sex hormones. Is a tonic for the uterus and its astringent power is used for excessive bleeding or hemorrhage. It is considered a specific for excessive blood loss during menopausal changes. It is mainly used for bleeding due to menses, fibroids and postpartum difficulties.

Black Haw

Actions - Astringent, antispasmodic, sedative, hypotensive, analgesic, uterine tonic.

Has a similar action to cramp bark to which it is closely related. Powerful relaxant of the uterus used for cramps and false labor pains. Can be used to prevent miscarriages. It can relax peripheral blood vessels thus reducing blood pressure. Its use for bleeding is confined to birthing and menopause.

Dong Quai

Actions - Emmenagogue, antispasmodic, analgesic, alterative, uterine tonic ,vasodilator.

Relieves some but not all of the symptoms of PMS and menopause by its action as a known regulator for the female reproductive system. Some of its compounds stimulate the uterus while others relax the uterus. The compounds that stimulate the uterus are water soluble and are absorbed into the body from teas and capsules. The compounds that relax the uterus are soluble in alcohol and are provided by tinctures. This herb may stop cramping, migraine attacks and eases the pain of ovarian cysts while there is less agreement on whether the herb stops hot flashes (wait and see after 6 weeks on the herb). The Chinese use this herb for abnormal menstruation, suppressed flow, painful or difficult menstruation.

Dose - 6 to 18 grams of dried root per day and in the tablet form 1500mg per day.

Note - This herb has a mild laxative effect. People who take blood thinners should avoid this herb.

Osteoporosis And Bone Pains

This disorder is characterized by a slow and progressive thinning and loss of the calcium content of the bones along with other minerals. Although the process actually begins in the fourth decade in both sexes it is accelerated in women after menopause. We all know the nasty things that can happen like hip fracture etc etc so I won't go into details. The first early warning signs of osteoporosis are those of calcium deficiency such as nocturnal leg cramps, joint pain, transparent skin, restless behavior and insomnia. In severe cases symptoms are very painful backache especially in the upper back. Always remember prevention is much easier then cure. Some medications interfere with calcium absorption; the ones to be weary of and to ask your pharmacist about are Corticosteroids, Anticonvulsants, Antacids containing aluminum and some Diuretics. The book now has a Acid and Alkaline Chart for the reason that excessively acid bodies try to make themselves more Alkaline so they tend to use what is easily available to do this which is usually Calcium and Magnesium which do a good job of buffering acid. Too much protein puts acid in the system, mainly uric acid which results from the breakdown of protein. Sugar put lots of acid in the body along with alcohol which when you break it down is just sugar. **Disease and Cancer are found in Acid bodies, it is said Cancer can't live in an Alkaline body.** Use alkaline foods to correct the imbalance. This is what the chart is for, it allows you to see if your diet is to acid and it shows you how to change it by eating more alkaline foods and reducing the acid foods.

High Risk Factors For Osteoporosis

1/. A diet high in animal protein
2/. Women who are light boned.

3/. Women who don't take enough exercise because they usually have low bone density.

4/. Women who have been on lots of punishing diets.

5/. Women who smoke as this brings on menopause earlier.

6/. Women who have a genetic predisposition to it ie mother has it.

7/. Poor unbalanced diet.

8/. Caffeine and alcohol encourage the excretion of calcium.

9/. Excessive salt intake makes our bodies excrete calcium and phosphorus which is another bone building mineral.

10/. Certain drugs increase the risk of osteoporosis examples are cortisone, thyroxine, tamoxifen, diuretics and antacids.

11/. Women who have had total hysterectomies including removal of their ovaries.

12/. Being underweight.

13/. Poor absorption of nutrients by the digestive system.

Nutrition For Osteoporosis

Calcium supplements are often poorly absorbed especially inorganic sources such as dolomite. Calcium should be combined with magnesium in the ratio of 2 to 1. A supplement should ideally contain other minerals and vitamins needed in the right proportions. Calcium taken alone depletes zinc and iron. Try a supplement that goes something like this 1000mg calcium,500mg magnesium, 10mg zinc, 3mg boron and a bit of Vitamin D. Take with it about 1000mg of vitamin C daily.

Even better try to get your calcium and minerals naturally from the diet, the only problem here is that only about 20 to 40% of calcium is absorbed and this gets worse with age. Vitamin D is needed for the absorption of calcium and for the body to make vitamin D it needs exposure to sunlight so make sure you get a bit of sun every day, go for a walk. Milk and other dairy products are not necessarily the best sources for natural calcium. Milk is low in magnesium which is needed to assimilate calcium and there are other foods that are higher. The table below suggests some other sources.

Boron - Boron is required for strong bones and the full absorption of calcium. Sources are apples, pears, grapes, dates, raisins, peaches, soybeans, almonds, hazelnuts, peanuts, honey. As a micro nutrient the dose is small about 1 to 2mg a day so a good dose is 2 apples and 3 and a half ounces of peanuts.

Calcium Rich Foods

Kelp (sea weed) per 100 grams	1093mg
Blackstrap molasses per 100 grams	579mg
Sardines per 100 grams	550mg
Dried figs per 100 grams	280mg
Almonds per 100 grams	250mg
Watercress per 100 grams	220mg
Sunflower seeds per 100 grams	100mg
Tofu per 100 grams	128mg

Comparison With Dairy Foods

Cow's milk per 100mls	120mg
Cheddar Cheese per 50 grams	400mg
Yogurt per 100 grams	180mg

Vaginal Changes

A variety of genital and urinary symptoms may develop on the way towards menopause as the lowering estrogen levels cause their changes. Falling estrogen levels cause the vaginal tissues to shrink along with atrophy and there is a loss of support due to the weakening of the pelvic tissues especially in women who have had many children, at the worst this might lead to prolapse.

The internal walls of the vagina thin and may become dry and sore and for some itchy.

Before the onset of menopause the thick walls of the vagina used to shed their skin cells and the harmless bacteria residing there would help turn this waste into lactic acid creating an acid environment which in turn protected the vagina from infections. Now that this has stopped the climate in the vagina has changed dramatically and it is unable to fend off invading bacteria as it used to. As a result offensive vaginal discharges are more common during the menopause and afterwards along with conditions such as cystitis. All these problems the dryness, thin walls, infections etc can cause pain on love making and not unnaturally put women off sex altogether. So what do we do? Well believe it or not regular sex and orgasm is the best way to keep the vagina in good working order. Lubrication has much less to do with the intensity of stimulation then with its duration so if you find yourself getting into difficulties share this information with your partner. Also another thing to remember is that in the post-menopausal women the clitoris is more exposed because of labial atrophy so this sensitive area becomes more vulnerable to stimulation which may be painful to some if the stimulation is to intense. If you find yourself losing interest in sex don't be too hard on yourself for it might be your balding partner with the big tummy just really doesn't turn you on anymore.

To gain an insight into how sex can keep the vagina in good health realize that every time you have an orgasm this pumps a massive amount of blood in the vagina which while it is there replenishes all the nutrients and takes away the wastes and add to this the old saying that covers every part of the body "use it or lose it".

Nutritional Treatment

Vitamin A and Beta Carotene help to sooth and heal the mucous membranes of the body.

Vitamin E is good for dryness of the vagina, and some skin problems.

Herbal Treatment

Black Cohosh is one of the main herbs for this and is taken internally usually in tincture, tea or pill form.

Vitex Agnus Castus - Is regarded throughout

Europe as the herb for menopause and PMS. It stimulates the pituitary (hormone control center) function altering FSH and LH secretions. Used for 3 months it will increase your levels of natural progesterone and help control hot flushes, depression and a dry vagina. Caution do not use with the birth control pill.

Wild Yam Progesterone Cream - Natural progesterone creams were used in the past for menopausal women who could not take estrogen and was found that in many cases it not only reversed osteoporosis but also reversed vaginal atrophying. If used with the herb above, Vitex could increase the internal progesterone output.

Some creams to think of that can be applied to the vagina are **Calendula Cream** which is antibiotic, anti-fungal, soothing and healing with another cream to think of being **Chick Weed** which is a specific for itching. I would be inclined to buy both of these creams and use calendula as the main one and mix Chick Weed with it only when relief from itching is needed.

Vaginal Changes And The Urinary System

The urinary track and the reproductive organs are located next to each other so what happens to one can affect the other. In menopause with the acid levels going down in the vagina the bacterial levels can go up increasing the possibility of urinary tract infections. Both the urinary tract and the reproductive organs rely on estrogen to function properly. Estrogen keeps the vagina moist and elastic keeping the tissues lubricated and flexible and the mucus membrane thick and productive. In its absence this all changes. Lack of estrogen affects the urethra by reducing the collagen and connective tissue that support the urethra which can make the tube inflexible and more easily damaged then it used to be, increasing the chance of bacterial invasion of the urinary system. This also makes it harder for the urethra to seal itself as well as it used to, adding to the chances of incontinence and increasing the chances of bacterial infection.

Urinary Tract Infections

Cause - A urinary tract infection (UTI) is an infection that begins in the urinary system. The urinary system includes the bladder, kidneys, ureters (the tube that carries urine from the kidney to the bladder) and the urethra (the tube that carries urine out of the body). An infection can be limited to the bladder; however, if the infection is not treated promptly, it can spread to the kidneys (called pyelonephritis) by travelling up the ureters, causing serious consequences. Urinary Tract Infection can infect anyone but women are more susceptible to this disease.

The main reason for the high incidence of bladder

infections in women is attributed to the shorter length of the urethra and its proximity to the vagina and the anal region, where the bacteria responsible for such infections are typically present. The condition is mainly caused when the bacteria from the digestive tract gets into the opening of the urethra. Sexual intercourse is another reason for urinary tract infections because the bacteria present in the vaginal tract is pushed inside the urethra. Having different sexual partners can be another reason for urinary tract infection. Waiting too long to urinate may also cause this infection. Prolonging urination causes stretches in the bladder. This stretching weakens the bladder not allowing it to completely empty itself. The urine which remains in the bladder increases your chances of the infection. Women who use a diaphragm may be more vulnerable to bladder infections, since the spermicide used with the diaphragm also suppresses the normal vaginal bacteria, upsetting the balance and allowing harmful bacteria to flourish. Post-menopausal women may be susceptible to bladder infections because of the effects of decreased oestrogen production as this can cause a thinning of the vaginal and vulvar tissues that are located around the urethra. One of the common urinary tract infections is bladder infection. Cystitis is the other name for bladder infection. Urethritis is the name of a condition when the infection occurs in the urethra while Pyelonephritis is the name of the condition when the infection occurs in the kidneys. This type of UTI requires urgent treatment, as it can lead to the malfunctioning of the kidneys and can also lead to death if not treated properly. A type of bacteria called Escherichia coli (E. coli) which normally lives in the colon is one of the major causes of most urinary tract infections. Chlamydia and Mycoplasma are some of the other micro-organisms that cause UTIs in both men and women. Usually these micro-organisms cause urinary tract infections in the urethra and reproductive system only.

The concentration of hydrogen-ion (commonly known as pH level) in the urinary tract defines how favourable the urine is for bacterial growth. On a scale of 0 to 14, a level of 7 is basic and neutral whereas a level of less that 7 is acidic. Researches and studies conducted to find the causes of bacterial growth point towards benefits of an alkaline pH in urine for preventing urinary tract infections and minerals, especially citrates, alkalise the urine. A steady dose of calcium or magnesium citrate supplements proves to be a great help in bladder infection treatment. As infected urine that remains in the bladder during the night can cause irritation to the bladder, mineral supplements should be taken at bedtime for better effect.

Chronic Urinary Infections - Infections that keep on recurring are often associated with yeast overgrowth. Candida overgrowth can be the main culprit and maybe mixed with this could be the onset of Diabetes which in turn makes the blood sweet which helps to feed the bacterial infection and also the Candida. An immediate treatment you could try is to recolonise the bowel with beneficial bacteria. Probiotic organisms are believed to compete with and crowd out the unhealthy organisms. Probiotic microorganisms such as Lacto-bacilli also make the bladder environment more acidic which in turn helps to prevent the growth of unwanted organisms. Try to find a Probiotic with as many strains as you can so as to try to repopulate as many beneficial strains as you can.

Prevention - If improperly treated, a urinary tract infection may spread to the kidneys. This can occur even though a person's symptoms appear to improve in one area. If there is any obstruction to the flow of urine because of bladder stones or because of enlargement of the prostate in men, there is an increase in the risk of bacteria remaining trapped in the bladder when they would normally be flushed out with urine. This causes a rapid build-up of bacteria and repeated bouts of bladder infections. So a good prevention for UTI infections would be to keep the urine alkaline and as soon as you become suspicious of an infection start to take a Cranberry supplement   immediately.

Symptoms - A very common symptom which UTI patients face through this condition is the constant urge to urinate. There will also be pain felt just above the pubic bone or radiating towards the lower back. Despite the presence of a constant urge to urinate there is a very minimal amount of urine passed. Urination is painful as well as leaves a burning sensation. The urine is also likely to be cloudy and have a stronger odour than usual.

You may suffer from fever if you have the infection in your kidneys. Bouts of vomiting and nausea are also possible. Backache and pain below your ribs are some of the other symptoms. Immediate treatment with antibiotics is necessary to prevent kidney damage and other serious consequences.

Prognosis - Continued infections lead to a risk of spread to the kidneys with maybe dangerous or have fatal consequences.

Treatment - Treatment if begun promptly is usually very effective and the condition should resolve within days or a week, depending on the severity of the infection. There is always the risk of recurrence however, which is why it is important that you continue the full course of medication prescribed by your doctor even if you feel better. It is very important for your system to have a good flow of urine. This can be done by consuming plenty of water. It cleanses your body by diluting and flushing out the unwanted substances. A mixture of 1/2 a teaspoon of baking soda in a eight ounce glass of water can be very helpful on the first signs of urinary tract infection as baking soda in your system can buffer the acidic urine. You can buy Alkalises from your chemist. You can maintain the alkaline content in urine by a rich diet in milk, fruits, and fresh vegetables.

Hot Compression Treatment -You can place a heating pad on the lower abdominal area to provide some relief to your pain. You can also use a hot water bottle but make sure that you refill it with hot water as soon as it starts to cool down. A hot compress not only helps to decrease inflammation but the extra heat helps to prevent the spread of the infection. Most bacteria and fungus require a warm condition to thrive but cannot survive in hot temperatures.

Herbal Treatment - Start with Cranberry (see below) to try to prevent the spread of the infection and also to shorten the duration. The main herbs we use in cystitis and UTIs are the Urinary Antiseptics with the best ones being Bearberry, Buchu and Goldenseal. To the Antiseptics we add Demulcents (see Actions Used In The Urinary System) which sooth the irritated tissues with the best one for this condition being Corn Silk, Marshmallow and also consider Licorice. You could add to the formula Gravel Root and Chaparral if you think the cause of the condition could be from urinary stones or gravel which tend to scratch and inflame the pipelines leaving them open to infection. Other herbs to consider are Angelica, Yarrow, Agrimony, Cleavers, Damiana, Horsetail, Golden Rod, Juniper, Plantain and Shepherds Purse. These herbs can be mixed as tinctures and most can be made into a tea. Always consider Echinacea in case the immune is down and also Zinc as this is the main mineral for the Reproductive and Immune Systems.

Cranberry

Constituents in cranberry called proanthocyanins

prevent bacteria from adhering to the walls of the urinary tract. This is thought to allow urine to wash away the bacteria. To put this in a easier to understand way, Cranberry lines the walls of the pipelines in the urinary system making it harder for bacteria to climb up them as it is slippery for them and lots of them keep getting washed away every time water is passed. If you have cystitis already this should protect the kidneys from infection especially at night when its just a downhill stroll for the bacteria. If you are using it as a preventative the lining on the urethra should hopefully protect the bladder. For best results use in 10.000mg doses morning and night.

Bearberry (Uva Ursi)

The active component, arbutin, appears to be broken down and then excreted in the kidneys, where it appears to have antiseptic properties. Uva ursi contains significant amounts of compounds called tannins. Tannins are not believed to be absorbed from the intestines. Tannins have an action of being antibacterial through their astringent properties. People with kidney, liver disease, pregnant, nursing women or children should not take Bearberry.

Treating Urinary Tract Infection by Aromatherapy

You can make an essential oil by using equal parts of sandalwood, bergamot, tea tree, frankincense and juniper. Mix all these ingredients to make an oil to be rubbed over your bladder area. Continue this massaging technique for three to four days once the symptoms subside.

Homoeopathic Treatment

Aconite 30C - People who are full of anxiety and fears, agitated and anxious at the thought of urinating because of the pain, frequent ineffectual and painful attempts to urinate, pain on pressure of bladder, may be blood in the urine. Condition may come on very fast. In the early febrile involvement when pulse and respiration are increased, symptoms worse by dry cold weather.

Apis 30C - Sharp stinging pains in lower abdomen with a frequent desire to urinate, intense pain, urine passes in small amount maybe with blood in it, the last few drops burn and smart, Renal edema in the acute form, urine shows albuminous casts. Heat makes all symptoms worse, improved by cold.

Belladonna 1M - Acute cases showing excitement and dilated pupils, full bounding pulse and hot smooth skin, straining to pass urine which is scanty and loaded with phosphates, blood in urine is common. There is a urge to try to urinate even after urine has passed. Dose every 2 hours for 4 doses.

Berberis 6C - Tenderness over the kidneys and sacral region accompanies frequent urination, the urine is cloudy and contains a reddish sediment. Dose 3 hourly for 4 doses.

Cantharis 30C - Much straining and scanty amounts of bloody urine, an unbearable urgency to urinate, cutting pain before, during and after urination, there is hyperexcitability and signs of sexual irritability, signs of abdominal pain prominent. Dose night and morning in chronic cases for one week, in acute cases give one dose every hour for 4 doses.

Causticum 30C - Great feeling of urgency to urinate but can be unable to, A useful remedy in the recurrent or chronic form and is especially adapted to older people. Follows well after Cantharis which may be needed if acute symptoms flare up in the chronic form. Very sensitive to cold.

Colocynthis 1M - Use for severe pain in the abdomen, the pains make patient double over. Signs of severe pain are present. Dose every hour for 4 doses.

Dulcamara 30C - Catarrhal cystitis resulting from exposure to cold or damp, urine contains a thick mucus or purulent sediment. Dose 3 times daily for 3 days.

Lycopodium 30C - A heavy feeling in the bladder mad better by holding abdomen, feels as if a ball is rolling around in bladder or lower abdomen, passes large volumes of urine at night and normal amounts during day. Urine profuse during the night, tendency to retention with thick reddish sediment. Dose night and morning for 5 days.

Mag Mur 6C - May help in preventing some forms of stones and may be given as a routine remedy if the urine shows suspicious deposits and there are other signs of stone formation.

Mercurius Sol 30C - Urine scanty with greenish mucous sediment which may contain pus and blood. Urine is dark colored. Dose 3 times daily for 4 days.

Nux Vom 30C - Pain before urination, sometimes

aborts urge to urinate. pain can be at the base of bladder with painful urination drop by drop. When ineffectual urging is associated with digestive upsets. Good to use if Cantharis does not work. Dose 3 times daily for 2 days.

Sarsaparilla 6C - Pain at the beginning and end of urination especially at the end, Urine contains gravely deposits and is slimy. Dose 3 times daily for 3 days.

Staphysagria 30C - Pressure upon the bladder, feels as if it did not empty, frequent urination, burning in urethra when not urinating, urging and pain after urinating. continual burning, result of sexual intercourse.

Urtica Urens 6X - Acid urine causes itching, itching and burning of the genitalia. Thickens the urine and removes the tendency to gravel formation by removing the basic salts that help form it, it will also increase the quantity of urine passed, there may be a skin rash, give one dose 3 times daily for 10 days.

Uva Ursi 3X - Useful in chronic cystitis, urine is slimy, pain and straining are common. Dose 3 times daily for 7 days.

Incontinence

When you can't hold back urine or it leaks out when you don't want it to you may be incontinent. Previous child bearing can play a great part in this condition or even surgery but the condition usually gets worse with the reduced amounts of estrogen which reduces flexibility and strength of the muscles surrounding the urethra.

Stress Incontinence – This is the most common form of incontinence where urine leaks when you laugh, cough or sneeze and is usually the result of child bearing or surgery with the added problem of less estrogen. The leakage occurs through pressure being put on the abdomen which in turn puts pressure on the bladder.

Treatment – Kegel exercises are a good way to strengthen the muscles around the urethra. (see below) Also think of Calc Flour in the Tissue Salts or Cell Salts as they are sometimes called as these are known as the elasticity salts as they put the springiness back in muscles and ligaments.

Urge Incontinence – This is where you feel a strong urge to urinate and can't make it to the bathroom or as the saying goes you get caught short. Spasms in the bladder cause this and it is usually a sign of another condition acting on the bladder. This needs a medical investigation to find the cause.

Kegel Exercises

Many factors can weaken your pelvic floor muscles, including pregnancy, childbirth, surgery, aging and being overweight. The purpose of these exercises is to strengthen the pubococcygeous muscles which are the ones that help you to stop urine from flowing. Step one is to identify these muscles as you need to exercise these alone. To identify the muscles try to stop urination in midstream. If you succeed, you've got the right muscles. Now that you have found them you are ready for the workout. Squeeze the muscles for about three seconds and then relax for five seconds repeat about five times trying to keep the other muscles relaxed. The best time to do this is when you go to the toilet to pass water as this way it's done constantly and you don't have to make a special time and place for the exercise.

The Cardiovascular System And Menopause

Estrogen is good for the cardiovascular system and protects you from, or really gives you about a ten year break from the problems that men have in this system with the worst being the Heart attack. Estrogen keeps the cardiovascular system healthy by lowering the blood pressure by dilating the blood vessels along with increasing the good cholesterol and lowering the bad. It also acts like an antioxidant helping to keep fat deposits from forming on the walls of your arteries and keeps the blood platelet from clotting too quickly. As the estrogen declines so does the protection to this system so now is a good time to re- evaluates your diet. Another piece of information that they don't tell you is that the female reproductive system uses about 500 calories a day so after menopause you require 500 calories a day less and to make matters worse the metabolism is slowing down which means fat will pass through the body slower giving the body a greater chance of absorbing all of it.

In later life heart disease is the biggest killer of women far greater than all the cancers put together. One of the main problems is that the symptoms of heart attack are different in woman then men. The crushing chest pains that men get in heart attack are not as common in women when they have a heart attack. The female pains are more like those of angina. For women, a heart attack is more likely to include some of the less classic symptoms such as nausea, abdominal pain, shortness of breath, and pain in the neck, shoulder or jaw. So female heart attack symptoms may not immediately make you think of the heart unless you are aware of the differences. Find out what your family history is like and that will give you the best clue of what you can expect.

Cardiovascular Risk Factors

Diet and Excessive Weight – As mentioned
before after menopause you will need 500 calories less per day then before, so if you eat what you always eaten you are going to put on weight. If you are overweight already then it's going to get a lot worse. So now is the time to start thinking about changing your diet for the better paying close attention to what your parents and close family health problems. Take time to work out a diet suitable for you and most importantly that you will enjoy.

Diabetes – What's your blood sugars like, has

anyone in the family got diabetes, are you a sweet tooth, now's the time to incorporate in your new diet diabetes prevention measures. Diabetes rapidly ages the cardiovascular system.

Cholesterol – After menopause the HDL (good cholesterol) levels begin to drop but a bigger change takes place with the LDL (bad cholesterol) as they start beginning to rise. Get your cholesterol checked and find out if anyone else in the family has cholesterol problems and make this another change for your diet.

Blood Pressure – Blood pressure is the force of blood against the walls of the arteries as it is circulated through the body. If the pressure in the arteries is too high the heart is forced to pump harder to force the blood through the body and as you can imagine this extra force leads to a lot of complications but unfortunately we usually do not find out till the damage is done because Hypertension is usually a symptomless condition.

What Causes High Blood Pressure - Although many different diseases can cause high blood pressure 90 percent of the time no cause is identified. This is known as Primary Hypertension. Some people have a greater risk of developing High Blood Pressure; the most common cause is being overweight. With a lot of people it runs in the family though in all of us our blood pressure will go up as we age. Other common causes are high salt intake, high alcohol intake, smoking and stress. Secondary

Hypertension is caused from a known disease with problems of the kidneys being one of the main causes though problems with the Endocrine system can also be a cause.

What Damage Does High Blood Pressure Cause - A lot of the damage is confined to the circulatory system, the first obvious problem occurs through the extra strain placed on the heart. Because the heart has to pump harder so as to force the blood through the vessels it becomes bigger and stronger but unfortunately it can get too big and when this happens it out grows its own blood supply and to make matters worse as the muscle grows it decreases the volume area in the heart, in other word the chambers inside the heart become smaller and the heart is now sending less blood into circulation. The inside of the blood vessels can be damaged by the excessive force of the flow of blood; this can lead to the onset of atherosclerosis which is the hardening and narrowing of the arteries. With the arteries narrowing the blood pressure increases and the condition gets worse leading to possible heart attack or strokes from a clot breaking free and blocking an artery or damage to the kidneys from a to high working pressure inside or the possibility of aneurysms which are a weak area in the artery ballooning out under the pressure and even possibly bursting.

How is High Blood Pressure Treated - Effective non drug treatments are a salt reduction in the diet, weight loss if overweight, improve your fitness, regular relaxation (relax twice a day for 20 minutes), reduce alcohol intake if you have more than 4 to 6 glasses a day, and stop smoking. If these measures don't have any effect or you need to get your blood pressure down immediately your Doctor will put you on Blood Pressure Lowering Drugs sometime for the rest of your life. Some of these drugs have side effects which you should discuss with your Doctor.

Alcohol – Women can't break down alcohol as fast as men so it tends to stay in the body longer. Three to four drinks a day will cause a noticeable rise in blood pressure. In large doses alcohol acts as a poison to the heart and that's not mentioning what it does to the poor liver.

Exercise – Now's the time to get the body back into shape not just for bone density reasons but because inactivity is the most common risk factor for heart disease in women. Exercise can lower the rate of heart disease by about 50% and don't forget that half of all women die from heart disease.

Herbal Treatment
Cleaning Out The Arteries

I always use Hawthorn and Ginkgo Biloba. Hawthorn is more the solvent to the plaques while Ginkgo opens up the arteries to let Hawthorn in to do its job. Both are antioxidants so we have doubled up on that action and have two herbs that help each other to get the job done. Do some research into both of these for they are the best team out for this condition?

Blood Pressure

I would use the two mentioned above mainly for all the other benefits. I have used Hawthorn with people already on blood pressure medication where it gives a slightly added drop in the blood pressure on top of the medication but generally in cases where the drugs have stopped keeping it sufficiently low. When doing this always monitor the result with a blood pressure machine and do it frequently. Blood pressure always works in waves, it will keep on rising for hours then it will drop so you have to do frequent readings to see if you are at the top of the wave or the bottom of the wave and work out an average. Hawthorn works like an adaptogen which means it tries to adapt you to your problems. If you have low blood pressure it raises it and if it is high it tries to lower it.

Two more herbs to consider or add to the mentioned herbs are Mistletoe and Lime Blossom. Mistletoe acts on the vagus nerve to reduce the heart rate and calms the nervous system and blood vessels while Lime Blossom is considered where stress and nervous tension is the main problems causing the problem.

Diet For Menopause

Now is the time for getting down or up to your right weight. In fact it would be better to stay just above your right weight so you have a bit of surplus fat helping in the making of estrogen. What you have to remember from now on is that you have the same risks for heart attack and all the other circulatory problems that males have. Another problem that we have to look out for is that we may not be absorbing our nutrients from food as good as we used to for the digestive system tends to be not as good as it used to be with digestive enzymes and acid becoming reduced. One way we can help to overcome this is to take digestive enzymes or take a glass of pineapple juice with our meals. A successful diet is more a change of lifestyle and has to be this way so as to keep the weight off.

1/. Have a high complex carbohydrate and low animal protein and fat diet. Complex carbohydrates are what their name implies they are complex so it takes a while to break down in digestion and this is good because it is releasing the sugars slowly which is what we want. Refined carbohydrates release their sugars fast which leads to high blood sugar then usually follows a slump of low blood sugar (hypoglycemia) and we all know high blood sugar causes diabetes.

2/. Elimination of refined sugar and refined flower products. Yes I know it's hard but you could do what I do and use honey as my main sweetener its good in coffee and as for refined flower, well we all know you can make glue using flower and water and this is what it does inside of you to as well as being responsible for most of the constipation people suffer from. Try to use unrefined preferably organic wholegrain products such as whole meal bread, whole meal flower for cakes, biscuits etc , whole meal pasta, brown rice.

3/. Cut back Caffeine - well at least give it a go. I am down to 1 cup of coffee a day now.

One of the problems here is that normally there is a lot of sugar with these products so cutting down in one helps with the other.

4/. Increase intake of green leafy vegetables to boost dietary fiber and mineral intake. Eat as much as possible of your fruits and veggies raw.

5/. Reduce salt intake, use vegetable salt instead of the normal table salt. If you suffer from fluid retention don't have any salt at all for the week after ovulation.

6/. Increase vegetable protein intake (nuts, beans and pulses including Soya products).

7/. If you are trying to lose weight have some protein with every meal. As mentioned before complex carbohydrates take a while for the digestive system to break down and protein is a lot more complex. This mixture should ensure that tummy is kept busy for a while and not asking for more.

8/. Increase consumption of essential fatty acids, dietary sources are found in raw nuts and seeds. Our Evening Primrose oil Supplement should cover most of this but see what you can do with the diet.

9/. Try to reduce your stress levels and start some form of exercise even if it's just a walk on the beach.

10/. Don't be too hard on your selves, give yourself your favorite meal on each 7th day and don't nag at yourself to much if you let yourself down just get up again and carry on the path.

If you follow a diet like this for life you would probably slowly reduce in weight, would reduce your chances of heart problems later in life, protect yourself from diabetes, have a good trouble free digestive system and be a very healthy person.

Diet And Nutrition For Menopause

There are plenty of foods and herbs that help in the production of hormone precursors which in turn help build hormones especially new estrogen. Support for the adrenal glands is very important for exhausted adrenals are not able to produce the hormones needed. For good adrenal function **Vitamin B Complex** and minerals including **Chromium** are required.

Less stress and more rest are imperative. Good liver function is of great importance as well so good care of the liver should be taken from now on. Changes in the parathyroid hormones means that metabolism of calcium is no longer efficient and it may be leached from the bones instead so high intakes in the minerals **Calcium** and **Magnesium** are needed from now on. Moderate exercise is even more important now, cycling and brisk walking which have been shown to preserve bone mineral density is particularly good.

Women from countries where naturally grown vegetables, seeds and fruits feature abundantly in the diet do not suffer from menopausal symptoms in the same way as those on western diets which tend to be high in protein but depleted in minerals. We eat far more protein then is necessary. Foods to avoid and cut down considerably include meat in particular, if you do eat it try to eat only organically reared meat that way you can escape from all the artificial hormones. Seafood is the ideal protein.

Also beware of sugar, coffee, chocolate, alcohol and any foods with chemical additives.

Following is a list of estrogenic foods and then we shall move on to diet.

Estrogenic Foods

Hormones are made in our bodies from the food we eat, below is a list of some of the most beneficial for menopause.

Seeds: Almost any sort, for example sesame seeds, pumpkin seeds, sunflower seeds, this includes sprouted seeds such as alfalfa, fenugreek, mung beans and lentils.

Wholegrains: Preferably organic - oats, wheat, rye, millet, buckwheat etc. These should be soaked then cooked whole. Add to salads or serve instead of rice.

Fresh Fruits: Bananas, avocados, papayas, mangoes.

Dried Fruits: Prunes, dates, figs, raisins, (all high in calcium).

Honey: Also bee pollen and Royal Jelly (be careful if you have allergies)

Culinary Herbs: Chervil, garlic, ginger, nutmeg, horseradish, sage, parsley, rosemary, Kelp.

Watercress and all dark green leafy vegetables are rich in minerals.

Cold Pressed Oils: Safflower is especially high in essential fatty acids, use this for cooking and adding to salads.

Nut Oils: Such as walnut and hazel nut, natural sources of Vitamin E and are essential for healthy skin and hair. Good for salad dressings.

Soybean Products: Only high protein soybean products have estrogenic activity that means soybeans, textured soy protein, tofu, soy milk and tempeh, but not soybean sauce and oil.

Phytoestrogen / Isoflavone Levels Of Soya Food

Soya Flakes – Half a cup = 130mg

Soya Flower – Half a cup = 85mg

TVP (Soya mince) – Half a cup = 70mg

Soya Beans Cooked – 100gms = 35mg

Soya Beans Sprouted – 100gms= 35mg

Tempeh – Half a cup = 35mg

Tofu (full fat) – 100gms = 30mg

Tofu (low Fat) – 100gms = 20mg

Soya Yoghurt – 100gms = 15mg

Soya milk (full Fat) – 1 cup = 10mg

Soya Milk (low fat) – 1 cup = 5mg

Miso – 1tbs = 5mg

Soya Cheese – 100mg = 3mg

Carbohydrates
Complex Carbohydrates
(Brown and Green foods)Lower in sugars, higher in nutrients

Whole meal bread
Brown rice
Brown pasta
Porridge oats
Muesli, Bran Cereals
Oatcakes, rye crackers
Jacket potato
Sweet Potato
Raw carrot, beets
Vegetable salads
Fibrous fruit

Simple Carbohydrates
(White Food) Higher in sugars lower in nutrients

White bread
White rice
White pasta
Instant oats
Cornflakes, Rice puffs
Water biscuits
Mashed or boiled potato
Most cakes and biscuits
Cooked carrots, parsnips and beets
Sugar

Alcohol

Calcium Rich Foods

Kelp (sea weed) per 100 grams	1093mg
Blackstrap molasses per 100 grams	579mg
Sardines per 100 grams	550mg
Dried figs per 100 grams	280mg
Almonds per 100 grams	250mg
Watercress per 100 grams	220mg
Sunflower seeds per 100 grams	100mg
Tofu per 100 grams	128mg

Comparison With Dairy Foods

Cow's milk per 100mls	120mg
Cheddar Cheese per 50 grams	400mg
Yogurt per 100 grams	180mg

Linda Kearns Hormone Cake
Menopause Cured The Yummy Way

In the 80s a women living in England by the name of Linda Kearns had been on hormone replacement therapy for 13 years following a hysterectomy along with the removal of her ovaries, but she had never really felt 100% with the treatment she was receiving as she always felt tired and a little under the weather. Latter Linda had a breast cancer scare, and we all know the link between HRT and breast cancer. Following the cancer scare she decided enough was enough and stopped taking the HRT.

Her hot flushes and night sweats soon appeared again so she began reading up on alternative therapies and discovered that she could replace the HRT using foods rich in phytoestrogens. The main problem was that a lot of these foods were not really appetizing, so she put her mind to the matter and decided to put the ingredients into a tasty cake. Within three weeks of starting to eat the cake her symptoms disappeared and she was bursting with energy. She now eats 2 slices of her cake every day at breakfast and after her evening meal.

About 100 grams (4oz) a day of the cake is usually enough to deliver a dose sufficient for the relief of menopausal problems. 100 grams looks big but it doesn't have to be eaten all at once and you don't have to worry about the sugar or fat content as there are no added fats other than those that occur naturally in the seeds and there is no added sugar in the cake.

Recipe For The Linda Kearns Cake
Ingredients
100g (4 oz) Soya Flower
100g Whole-wheat Flower
100g Porridge Oats
100g Linseeds
100g Sunflower Seeds
50G (2oz) Sunflower Seeds
50g Pumpkin Seeds
50g Sesame Seeds
50g Flaked Almonds
2 pieces of stem ginger finely cut
200g (8 oz) Raisins
Approx. 750 ml of Soya Milk
1 Tablespoon of malt extract
Half teaspoon of Nutmeg
Half teaspoon of Cinnamon
Half teaspoon ground ginger

Place the dry ingredients in a large bowl and mix thoroughly, then add the Soya Milk and Malt Extract. Mix well and leave to soak for about half an hour. If the mixture is to stiff add more Soya milk. Spoon into 2 loaf tins lined with grease proof paper and oil. Bake in the oven at 190 Celsius or 375 F for about 75 minutes or until cooked through (test with a skewer). Turn out and leave to cool. The cake goes well with butter or spread.

Nutrition For The Reproductive System

The 5 star Super Foods

Seeds especially pumpkin and sesame

Oats

Avocado

Walnuts

Extra Virgin Olive Oil

Celery

Bananas

The Super Foods

Fruits - Dates. pineapple, citrus fruits, cherries ,blackcurrants, strawberries, rosehips, olives, apricots, peaches.

Vegetables - Carrots, dark green vegetables, onions, avocado, nettles.

Grains - Maze, oats, whole wheat bread, wheat germ, buckwheat, millet, rye flower.

Pulses - Soybeans, lentils, peas, beans.

Nuts and Seeds - Alfalfa, sprouted seeds, mung beans, soy beans, almonds, hazelnuts, peanuts, cashew nuts.

Herbs and Spices - Parsley, peppermint, fenugreek, sage.

Others - Cold pressed sunflower oil, oily fish, cod liver oil, cheeses, butter, brewer's yeast, molasses, honey, pollen eggs, oysters and shellfish.

The Danger Foods

Fats - In excess, old and rancid fats or foods cooked in them.

Refined Carbohydrates - White flour and sugar deplete levels of B vitamins they are also a heavy tax on the digestive system which drains vital energy. Avoid processed foods.

Meat - Choose organic and free range meat and poultry to avoid the possible ingestion of chemicals from animal medicines and treated animal feed. Sea food is good.

Tonic Herbs For This System - Female - Black haw, Damiana, Dong Quai, Siberian Ginseng, Squaw vine, Liquorices.

Cancer And Breast Cancer

Cancer is our modern day epidemic disease, if you live to a good old age and survive everything else you will either die of heart disease or cancer. In a healthy person cells divide, grow and replace them in an ordinary way. When the gene that controls normal cell function fails from a variety of reasons such as age, improper nutrition, stress or toxic burden, the cell becomes sick and starts dividing and multiplying out of control. A mass of these uncontrolled cells are called a tumor. Some of these tumors eventually stop growing and are considered benign (harmless). Malignant tumors however continue to grow and eventually invade healthy tissues and use up the bodies nutritional stores and disrupt body functions. Hormonal cancer of the breasts, ovaries and prostrate are very common. 40% of breast cancers are in women under the age of 60. From 60 years of age the percentage increases to 60%. You have a higher risk of breast cancer if it has happened before in your family or if you started your periods at a young age such as 10 and came to your menopause late at about 59. If you have not had children or had them late in life is another risk factor along with a history of benign breast disease.

Modern genetic research has identified several genes that increase the risk of breast cancer, but at present there are only tests for two of them, BRCA1 and BRCA2. Your risk of getting breast cancer if you carry either of these genes is about 85% by the time you are

55 years old.

Although many of the risk factors for breast cancer are beyond your control, you can still take steps to decrease your risk by changing your diet and eating lots more fresh fruit, bran cereals, whole meal bread and raw salads daily. This will increase the roughage in the diet which will help to protect you from cholesterol and bowel cancer along with upping your vitamin and mineral uptake which should also give you a protective antioxidant action. 35% of cancers are directly related to poor nutrition. Also keep an eye on alcohol consumption as there is a relation between it and cancer. Always think of prevention by checking the breasts regularly and at least one mammogram a year, if you are in the high risk category get one every six months. The earlier breast cancer is detected the more effectively it can be treated.

Most cancers today would be greatly reduced if our environment was not so contaminated. Most of us are exposed to harmful chemicals, industrial carcinogens, and solvents present in cleaning solutions, cosmetics, pesticides, plastics and processed foods. Two documented but little known risk factors for ovarian cancer are dying your hair regularly and using prescription antidepressants. Breast cancer risks include being overweight, lack of regular exercise, environmental pollution, using prescription hormones and wearing ill-fitting bras.

Flaxseeds - Several studies have shown the regular

ingestion of flaxseeds will lower the estrogen that promotes tumor growth in the breasts.

Translucent Light Breast Lump Check For Remote Areas

If you live in a remote area without many medical facilities and you detect a lump in your breast or a friend does you can do what they used to do which is get a good torch and find a darkened room or even better wait till night then put the torch under the breast or sit the breast on the torch in the area the lump was found and turn the torch on. With the light shining through the breast you should be able to see the lump. When you see the lump and make out the shape but see that the light is still going through the area it usually means the area is filled with fluid, but if you see the lump and no light passes through it then it is probably a solid mass in which case it could be a tumor.

Introducing the Acid and Alkaline Chart

I now believe one of the main causes of cancer is from the body being constantly acidic. It is said **Disease and Cancer are found in Acid bodies, it is said Cancer can't live in an alkaline body.** My training as an Iridologist taught me to see what acid eyes look like and the constant contacts of people with cancer over the years slowly lead me to this conclusion. So a long time ago I made my own Acid and Alkaline Chart as it was the only way I could get one at the time. For over a decade everyone with cancer was shown the chart and we tried to work out where their diet was and nearly all the time they were in the acid areas of the chart or as I refer to it in the acid lane or living in the acid lane. . Recently I was in a very large Pharmacy in the middle of a state capital city for a few years where I had dealings with literally thousands of people with lots of them being tourists. Anyone with cancer was shown the chart and had it explained to them with the result of most of them being in the acid lane not only in food but usually from stress, worry and overwork. Anger also raises the acid levels and I have seen many who are angry and now even more angry that their body has betrayed them and who's going to look after my young family now. They stand in front of me with their fists clenched tight and you can almost feel the rage, this is not fair, it's not right, what am I going to do, who will look after my family. Using this as an example you can see why you have to remove the cause. You have to explain to them what their rage and diet is doing to them. Someone with that amount of anger and stress is rapidly using up all their B vitamins along with calcium and magnesium which the nervous system would be gobbling up at a fast rate as its taking most of the burden from the stress and then imagine how much adrenaline must be in the blood of one so angry so that's more B vitamins are being used to support that system. Let's move this case further along and see what else is happening. Human blood is always slightly alkaline if it goes into the acid we die of what is called Acidosis. So if you are living in the acid lane and your blood is in a constant battle to keep itself in the alkaline lane then the body is in constant stress which makes more acid, but it has no choice but to keep it self-alkaline so to do that it has to use the minerals in the body to buffer that acid with the main ones being Calcium and Magnesium. So imagine a lifetime in the acid lane living on processed food and fizzy drinks which are pumped full of carbonic acid to make the bubbles and loaded with sugar which breaks down to acid and you get the sad picture of lots of people with cancer and lots of people with osteoporosis because the blood has had to steal its Calcium and Magnesium from the bones because it's taken it from every other place as much as it can without breaking down the system. Sometimes the chemist has sent over to me people with cancer who are obviously close to the end of their time and I have shown them the chart, explained it and then given them a photocopy of it and a couple of months later they will pop up and come and see me and say they think it has helped them a bit.

Guide To The Chart

Excessively acid bodies try to make themselves more Alkaline so they tend to use what is easily available to do this which is usually Calcium and Magnesium which do a good job of buffering acid. Too much protein puts acid in the system, mainly uric acid which results from the breakdown of protein. Sugar put lots of acid in the body along with alcohol which when you break it down is just sugar. **Disease and Cancer are found in Acid bodies, it is said Cancer can't live in an Alkaline body.** Use alkaline foods to correct the imbalance. This is what the chart is for, it allows you to see if your diet is to acid and it shows you how to change it by eating more alkaline foods and reducing the acid foods.

1. - **Human blood pH should be slightly alkaline (7.35 - 7.45). A pH of 7.0 is neutral. A pH below 7.0 is acidic. A pH above 7.0 is alkaline. A blood pH of 6.9, which is only slightly acidic, can induce coma and death.**

2. - **An acidic pH can occur from, an acid forming diet, emotional stress, toxic overload, immune reactions or any process that deprives the cells of oxygen and other nutrients. The body will try to compensate for acidic pH by using alkaline minerals. If the diet does not contain enough minerals to compensate, a buildup of acids in the cells will occur.**

3. - **Alkaline or Acid forming describes ash residue after metabolism. Citrus tastes acidic but leaves an alkaline residue.**

4. - **Disease and Cancer are found in Acid bodies, it is said Cancer can't live in an Alkaline body. Use alkaline foods to correct the imbalance.**

5. - **Most people eat acid producing processed foods**

like white flour and sugar and drink acid producing beverages like coffee and soft drinks. We use too many drugs, which are acid forming; and we use artificial sweeteners.

6. - To maintain health, the diet should consist of 60% alkaline forming foods and 40% acid forming foods. To restore health, the diet should consist of 80% alkaline forming foods and 20% acid forming foods.

7. - Generally, alkaline forming foods include: most fruits, green vegetables, peas, beans, lentils, spices, herbs and seasonings, and seeds and nuts.

8. - Generally, acid forming foods include: meat, fish, poultry, eggs, grains, and legumes.

9. - Protein foods combine well with vegetables but not starches. Starches combine well with other vegetables and also light protein such as dairy foods.

10. - Fruit is best on its own. For digestive distress use Lemon juice as this is a great alkalizer.

11. - Try to make the diet 80% alkaline and 20% acid when you start using the chart. Lemon can be added to sauces, casseroles and fish to reduce acid. Nibble on dates etc.

12. - Add lemon juice to the fridge cold water so every time you drink it you are alkalizing the body.

13. - Rest, sleep and exercise are all alkalizers while the negative emotions make acid. Remember to eat according to you occupation.

14. - Deep breathing releases at least 50% of body toxins so set a time aside each day to do this for a

while. Remember happy cells don't mutate.

Herbs - Some of the best herbal digestive remedies are Ginger, Peppermint, Chamomile and Dandelion; these can be had in a tea. Apple Cider Vinegar or Lemon can be added to the teas for their alkalizing effect. Foods can be cooked with herbs for those with poor tummies. Think of the mentioned herbs and then add Fennel, Anise, Cayenne, dill, Garlic, Parsley. Fenugreek, Curry etc. See an Herbalist for Herbs more suited to your condition.

The Acid And Alkaline Chart

For protection against Cancer and Osteoporosis use the Acid and Alkaline Chart. Excessively acid bodies try to make themselves more Alkaline so they tend to use what is easily available to do this which is usually Calcium and Magnesium which do a good job of buffering acid. Too much protein puts acid in the system, mainly uric acid which results from the breakdown of protein. Sugar put lots of acid in the body along with alcohol which when you break it down is just sugar. **Disease and Cancer are found in Acid bodies, it is said Cancer can't live in an Alkaline body.** Use alkaline foods to correct the imbalance. This is what the chart is for, it allows you to see if your diet is to acid and it shows you how to change it by eating more alkaline foods and reducing the acid foods. Diet is very important, consider this, every 3 months the blood replaces itself, every year the bones replace themselves. In a year's time are you going to have a healthy body or a junk food body with McDonald bones. Don't forget if you eat on the acid side the bones won't be all that strong anyway.

Extremely Acid Forming Foods - pH 5.0 to 5.5

5.0 - Artificial sweeteners, Overwork, Fear, Stress, Anger, Jealously.

5.5 - Beef, Carbonated soft drinks & fizzy drinks, Cigarettes (tailor made), Drugs, Flour (white, wheat), Goat, Lamb, Pastries & cakes from white flour, Pork, Sugar (white), Beer, Brown sugar, Chicken, Deer, Chocolate, Coffee, Custard with white sugar, Jams, Jellies, Liquor, Pasta (white), Rabbit, Semolina, Table salt refined and iodized, Tea black, Turkey, Wheat bread, White rice, White vinegar (processed).

Moderate Acid - pH 6.0 to 6.5

6.0.-.Cigarette tobacco (roll your own), Fish, Fruit juices with sugar, Maple syrup (processed), Molasses (sulphured), Pickles (commercial), Breads (refined) of corn, oats, rice & rye, Cereals (refined) e.g. Weetabix, corn flakes, Shellfish, Wheat germ, Whole Wheat foods, Wine, Yogurt (sweetened)

6.5 - Bananas (green), Buckwheat, Cheeses (sharp), Corn & rice breads, Egg whole (cooked hard), Ketchup, Mayonnaise, Oats, Pasta (whole grain), Pastry (wholegrain & honey), Peanuts, Potatoes (with no skins), Popcorn (with salt & butter), Rice (basmati), Rice (brown), Soy sauce (commercial), Tapioca, Wheat bread (sprouted organic)

Slightly Acid to Neutral pH 7.0

7.0 - Barley malt syrup, Barley, Bran, Cashews, Cereals, (unrefined with honey-fruit-maple syrup),

Cornmeal, Cranberries, Fructose, Honey (pasteurized), Lentils, Macadamias, Maple syrup (unprocessed), Milk (homogenized) and most processed dairy products, Molasses (unsulphered organic), Nutmeg, Mustard, Pistachios, Popcorn & butter, (plain), Rice or wheat crackers (unrefined), Rye,(grain), Rye bread (organic sprouted), Seeds, (pumpkin & sunflower), Walnuts, Blueberries, Brazil nuts, Butter (salted), Cheeses, (mild & crumbly), Crackers (unrefined rye), Dried beans, Dry coconut, Egg whites, Goats milk (homogenized), Olives (pickled), Pecans, Plums, Prunes.

Slightly Alkaline to Neutral pH 7.0

7.0 – Almonds, Artichokes (Jerusalem), Barley-Malt, Brown Rice Syrup, Brussels Sprouts, Cherries, Coconut (fresh), Cucumbers, Eggplant, Honey (raw), Leeks, Miso, Mushrooms, Okra, Olives ripe, Onions, Pickles, (homemade), Radish, Sea salt, Spices, Taro, Tomatoes, (sweet), Vinegar (sweet brown rice), Water Chestnut, Artichoke (globe), Chestnuts (dry roasted), Egg yolks (soft cooked), Goat's milk and whey (raw), Horseradish, Mayonnaise (homemade), Millet, Olive oil, Rhubarb, Sesame seeds (whole), Soy beans (dry), Soy cheese, Soy milk, Sprouted grains, Tempeh, Tofu, Tomatoes (less sweet), Yeast, (nutritional flakes)

Moderate Alkaline - pH 7.5 to 8.0

8.0 - Apples (sweet), Apricots, Alfalfa sprouts, Arrowroot, Flour, Avocados, Bananas (ripe), Berries, Carrots, Celery, Currants, Dates & figs, (fresh), Garlic, Gooseberry, Grapes (less sweet), Grapefruit, Guavas, Herbs (leafy green), Lettuce, (leafy green), Nectarine, Peaches (sweet), Pears, (less sweet), Peas (fresh sweet), Pumpkin (sweet), Sea salt (vegetable), Spinach

7.5 - Apples (sour), Bamboo shoots, Beans (fresh green), Beets, Bell Pepper, Broccoli, Cabbage; Cauliflower, Carob, Daikon, Ginger (fresh), Grapes (sour), Kale, Lettuce (pale green), Oranges, Parsnip, Peaches (less sweet), Peas (less sweet), Potatoes & skin, Pumpkin (less sweet), Raspberry, Strawberry, Squash, Sweet corn (fresh), Tamari, Turnip, Vinegar (apple cider)

Extremely Alkaline Forming Foods - pH 8.5 to 9.0

8.5 - Agar, Cantaloupe, Cayenne (Capsicum), Dried dates & figs, Kelp, Limes, Mango, Melons, Papaya, Parsley, Seedless grapes, (sweet), Watercress, Seaweeds, Asparagus, Endive, Kiwifruit, Fruit juices, Grapes (sweet), Passion fruit, Pears (sweet), Pineapple, Raisins, Vegetable juices

9.0 – Lemons, Watermelon.

Nutrition For Cancer

The 5 star Super Foods

Apricots

Beetroot

Cabbage

Carrots

Garlic

The Super Foods

Fruits - Apples, apricots, bananas, all citrus fruits, all the berries particularly cranberries, cantaloupe, melons, yellow peaches, strawberries, persimmons.

Vegetables - Asparagus, endives, cabbage, broccoli, Brussels sprouts, cauliflower, horseradish, kale, mustard, radishes, turnips, watercress, lettuce, mushrooms, red yellow and green peppers, potatoes, pumpkins, sweet potatoes, yams.

Grains - Barley, brown rice, buckwheat, millet, whole-wheat and wheat germ.

Dried Fruit - Apricots and prunes.

Pulses - Lentils, chickpeas, all the beans.

Seeds and Nuts - Almonds, hazelnuts, pumpkin, sesame and sunflower seeds, walnuts.

Herbs - Parsley, garlic, chamomile, thyme, cloves, sage, rosemary.

Others - Extra virgin olive oil, fermented foods and liquids - yoghurt, quark, sauerkraut.

Drinks - Fermented fruit and vegetable juices especially beetroot, cabbage, carrot and potatoes, papaya juice, pineapple juice.

The Danger Foods

Animal Protein - High meat intake has been associated with high incidence of cancer particularly of the bowel, pancreas and prostrate.

Rancid Fats Oils and Nuts - Harmful free radicals are produced when oily foods oxidize or turn rancid.

Saturated Fats - Fat is one of the major dietary promoters of cancer.

Smoked ,Barbecued and Salt Cured Foods - Bacon, kippers, pickled herrings, vegetables in brine, charcoal grilled steaks all contain carcinogenic substances.

Processed Meat - Products persevered with nitrites and nitrates are high in salt and saturated fat, such as salami, sausages, ham, luncheon etc and should be avoided as nitrites are converted in the stomach into nitrosamines which are highly carcinogenic.

Mouldy Food - The moulds that form on some foods are carcinogenic.

Supplements For Menopause

Vitamins

1/. **Vitamin A** and Beta Carotene help to sooth and heal the mucous membranes of the body. Vitamin A can also reduce excessive bleeding and thus help prevent anemia.
Food Sources - Apricots, carrots, green leafy vegetables, liver, mint, egg yolk.

2/. **Cod Liver Oil** - Good sources of vitamins A and D. You need vitamin D and sunlight for the assimilation of calcium.

3/. **B 5** Important for proper adrenal gland function. Sometimes a deficiency shows up as anxiety attacks, burning feet and abdominal attacks.

4/. **Vitamin B6 (Pyridoxine).** A number of studies have found that B6 in a daily dosage of 25 to 100mg can give satisfactory relief too many PMS symptoms such as premenstrual headaches, fluid retention, irritability, mood swings and depression in around 60 to 80% of women. B6 helps to regulate the brains biochemistry and is necessary for the conversion of tryptophan to the brain hormone serotonin. Serotonin is a natural regulator of mood, sex drive, sleep and appetite. B6 helps prevent anemia.

Food Sources - Brewer's yeast, raw nuts and seeds, pith of citrus fruits (marmalade).

5/. **B 12** can also be of benefit. It may be a good idea to buy B6 and B12 and use them by themselves for a while or at least a container full so you can observe the effect on yourself.

B12 and **Folic acid** can help to improve energy levels and prevent anemia. If fatigue and or depression is a problem take 250 to 500micrograms of B12 and 800micrograms of Folic Acid daily.

Food Sources - Clams, egg yolk, herring, liver, meat, milk, oysters, salmon, sardines.

6/. **B Complex** - As most of the Bs work together it can be easier and cheaper just to take a complex formula. This complex is good for the nerves and adrenal glands.

7/. **Hesperidin or Bioflavonoids** - Bioflavonoids have been used successfully to reduce hot flashes as well as to reduce heavy bleeding. They also help protect and strengthen capillary walls. This helps to reduce hot flashes by improving venous tone, restoring normal capillary permeability and improving lymphatic drainage. Take 500mgs 3 times daily with 500mgs of Vitamin C as long as you have symptoms. The main bioflavonoids are rutin, quercetin, citrin, hesperidin, genestein and diadzein.

Food Sources - Buck wheat, citrus fruit, sprouts, skins of fruits, vegetables and soy products.

8/. Vitamin E - Involved in the production of some of the pituitary and adrenal hormones. In the 1940s women with cancer or prone to cancer were given vitamin E with good results that were well documented because they couldn't use oestrogen because of their cancer risk. Vitamin E is a hormone normalizer. Tests have shown that when E is low the levels of FSH and LH increase. As these levels are high anyway in women going through menopause a lack of E could make the problem far worse. Helps to alleviate hot flashes, breast tenderness and other menopausal problems, is a very potent anti-oxidant, other menopausal problems E can help with are excessive or scanty periods, nervousness, fatigue, insomnia, dizziness, heart palpations, shortness of breath reduced sexual desire, dryness of the vagina, and some skin problems.

Food sources - Wheat germ oil and all cold pressed oils from vegetable sources, sesame seeds, sunflower and pumpkin seeds, hazel nuts, walnuts, peanuts, sprouted seeds, spinach, Brussels sprouts, brown rice, asparagus, celery, peas, avocado.

Caution - No one taking anticoagulant drugs for thrombosis or other similar conditions should take Vitamin E.

Minerals

1/. Boron - Eating foods rich in the micro mineral Boron can boost estrogen levels and boron is required for strong bones and the full absorption of calcium. Sources are apples, pears, grapes, dates, raisins, peaches, soybeans, almonds, hazelnuts, peanuts, honey. As a micro nutrient the dose is small about 1 to 2mg a day so a good dose is 2 apples and 3 and a half ounces of peanuts.

2/.Calcium - Calcium supplements are often poorly absorbed especially inorganic sources such as dolomite. Calcium should be combined with magnesium in the ratio of 2 to 1. A supplement should ideally contain other minerals and vitamins needed in the right proportions. Calcium taken alone depletes zinc and iron. Try a supplement that goes something like this 1000mg calcium, 500mg magnesium, 20mg zinc, 3mg boron and about 1000mg of vitamin C daily.

3/. Chromium - Helps to improve efficient use of insulin and keep blood sugar levels steady. Take 100 to 200 micrograms once or twice a day.

Food Sources - Asparagus, grape juice, prunes, raisins, nuts, mushrooms, molasses.

4/. Magnesium - This mineral is often deficient in women who consume a diet that is high in refined carbohydrates and sugar. Such diets deplete the body of the minerals chromium, manganese, zinc ,magnesium and the B complex vitamins. Women with PMS have been found to have lower levels of magnesium in there red blood cells compared to unaffected women.

Women with magnesium deficiency often crave sugar

and in particular chocolate.

Magnesium is a very important mineral for the nervous system and a deficiency can cause cramps. Perimenopausaul symptoms caused by magnesium deficiency can be nervousness, anxiety, irritability, cramps, tremors, concentration problems, apathy and depression.

Food sources - lettuce, garlic, tomatoes, potatoes, raisins, bananas, almonds, cashews, dates, most whole grains, wheat germ, spinach, peas, celery.

5/.Zinc - Commonly deficient in the western diet. Zinc is necessary for the proper functioning of the ovaries and the reproductive system in both sexes and is also needed for the immune system. 15 to 50mg per day helps to lower estrogen and increase progesterone levels which can help perimenopausaul women. It promotes strong and healthy skin and hair and helps in wound healing and bone formation.

Food sources - Rose hip tea, brewer's yeast, wheat germ, pumpkin seeds, egg yolk and oysters, now you know why oysters are meant to be a aphrodisiac.

Amino Acids

1/. Tryptophan (Amino Acid) - Women with flushes and night sweats can have their symptoms relieved by taking 500mg in fruit juice before sleep. Low levels of this are associated with anxiety and insomnia in menopausal women. The types of depression that can be treated with Tryptophan are usually associated with cravings for carbohydrates.

Food sources - Cottage cheese, soybean, fish, lintels, peanuts, pumpkin seeds, sesame seeds.

2/.Glutamine (**Amino Acid**) - Helps to improve mental clarity, fatigue, reduces blood sugar, reduces sugar cravings, alleviates aggressiveness, improves mood, improves concentration and lifts depression. Take 500 to 1000mg twice daily for 3 months.

Food Sources - Papaya, celery, parsley, spinach, cabbage, lettuce, carrots and Brussels sprouts.

Essential Oils For The Diet

Evening Primrose Oil - This is the most important supplement out of the lot. A lot of people have found that just taking this and B6 can get rid of their problems. EPO (Evening Primrose Oil) is an essential fatty acid and here we are using it to balance the prostaglandin families. What we are trying to do is replace the bad fats with the good ones. EPO increases the good prostaglandins and can be remarkably effective in reducing premenstrual headaches, arthritis, breast tenderness, period pains and other symptoms of PMS. EPO is helpful for ovarian function and helps to return regularity to the menstrual cycle and can also reduce ovarian cysts and ease any pains and inflammations. Try taking about 3 x 1000mlg oil capsules a day. Sometimes you have to take this for a few months to gain the full benefit.

Flax Seed Oil - Contains both Omega 3 and 6 fatty

acids. Because it helps to balance estrogen Flaxseed oil is a good remedy for prerimenopausal symptoms especially skin conditions, depression and fatigue. It also fights cancer, lowers cholesterol levels and makes insulin more effective. This oil also discourages the body from storing fat, enhances the immune system and reduces the risk of osteoporosis.

Fish Oil Omega 3 - Our brains are mostly made of fat and this is one fat that the brain really needs. We can't produce Omega 3 so we must get it from external sources with the best being cold water fish such as salmon and tuna. The only plant source of Omega 3 is Flaxseed oil.

Exercise

Exercise is very important, with one of the main reasons being to build up your bone density while you still have a chance and the cardio vascular improvements could also reduce hot flushes and many other symptoms brought on by perimenopause. One hour of moderate exercise five times a week will improve your health and the quality of your life. Lower estrogen levels can contribute to a number of medical conditions, memory lapses and emotional transformations. Physical activity can help you reclaim your grip on life and help fight off cardiovascular disease, diabetes, cancer, osteoporosis, loss of muscle tone and strength and helps control your weight and emotional wellbeing as well as giving you increased self-esteem.

A good fitness plan has been shown to relieve anxiety, irritably, mood swings, decreased libido and depression and by sticking to the plan you have time to build your physical fitness as well as your emotional fitness.

It has been found that in woman who exercise only 1 in 20 get hot flushes compared to 1 in 4 who don't. Exercise also improves your sleep by not only making you more tired but also by increasing the levels of melatonin a natural hormone that helps regulate sleep. Best of all exercise is the one supplement that you can take that costs no money and gives you more benefit then taking lots of supplements. You may wish to consider one of the adaptogen herbs such as Maca to make it easier for you to get started and also to improve your energy levels at the beginning.

Introduction to Herbal Medicine

Herbal Medicine has been in use and developed continuously since the beginning of time. It mainly evolved from observations from what plants did and the affects they had on people along with their animals. There is also what they call the Doctrine of Signatures which works like this, that flower really looks like an eye, maybe it helps sore eyes? I'll give it a try as my eyes are so sore and red. You know my eye really feels a lot better now, I think I will call that plant Eye Bright (Euphrasia) and tell my friends all about it especially my Dad who gets sore eyes to. In this way hundreds of plants were identified that have a medical action and no doubt there were also a lot of casualties. The next great leap in herbal medicine was the Roman Empire of 2000 years ago. The Great Armies of Rome all had their own Medical Corps with Doctors, Battle Surgeons and Orderlies. It was these men who already had the knowledge of the Greeks that started to put together the best medical manuals in the world while at the same time started developing and using medical instruments and tools some of which are still used today. As the Romans conquered the known world more medicines and knowledge were found and assimilated. The next great leap was modern Chemistry which allowed us to see exactly what herbs were made up of and what parts of the herb causes its medical action. Drug companies have made billions of Dollars from this information as they find the main active ingredient and then make a synthetic version of it, one good example that we all know of is Valium which is the synthetic version of the active ingredient from the herb Valerian. Leaving aside the Drug Companies let's see how Chemistry changed the way that modern herbalists think. Modern science allows us to now know what Actions our herbs perform on the body so we shall carry on using Valerian as a example and see what Medical Actions Valerian has on the body. The Actions of Valerian are Sedative, Hypnotic (sleep inducing), Anti Spasmodic (stops twitches, cramps etc.), Hypotensive (lowers Blood Pressure) and Carminative (calms and relaxes the tummy). Herbalists call Valerian the Herbal Tranquillizer and if you look at the actions you can see why for if you can't sleep and your blood pressures up along with a gurgling tummy and an eye constantly twitching you definitely need to be calmed down. The modern herbalist is trained to think in actions. There are many reasons for this but the main ones are to stop them from just using a handful of their favorite herbs and to train the mind to work in the method of thinking in actions that are needed. If we start thinking in the actions that are needed for a patient it makes us consider the problem in far more depth than just using our favorite herb and it forces our thinking to be far more holistic by taking in consideration the whole of the patient not just the part or the system we wish to treat. Let's take a look at thinking in actions.

The patient has a cough, but when coughs can't stop and the cough sounds a bit like whooping cough. The patient also sounds a little hoarse and the temperature is also elevated. The actions that come into mind for this are expectorant for the cough, antispasmodics for the whooping quality of the cough and demulcents to sooth the sore throat. These are the obvious actions and we can add many more if we wish such as immune boosters for acute diseases, diaphoretics to reduce the temperature and prevent a fever and the list goes on. Next we look at how Herbal Actions are used in making Herbal Formulas. Another point to make before we go to the formula making is that Professional Herbalists use Herbs in the form of Tinctures (water and alcohol solutions) as this allows them to mix formulas in any proportions that they like and also allows long term storage without spoiling.

Making Herbal Formulas

You should never have more the 5 Herbs in a herbal formula otherwise you start to lose track of what you are doing and how the formula is changing the symptoms. Always try to keep things simple. One of the herbs in the formula is used to force the formula into the body, to keep it simple we will only use three, they are Licorice, Ginger and Cayenne. As an example let's use a patient with a cough. After further study of the case we decide that this is an Acute Disease for it came on quickly and is fast acting not slow like a

Chronic Disease. Listening to the patients cough we decide that it is a dry cough and the patient has not got a runny nose. Let's list the actions to consider.

Expectorants - Licorice, Aniseed, Fennel, Garlic and Mullein

Antispasmodics - Aniseed and Fennel

Demulcents - Licorice and Coltsfoot

Immune Boosters - Echinacea

Anti-Bacterial and Virals - Garlic and Echinacea

Out of the above I would choose Licorice, Echinacea, Garlic, Aniseed and Fennel. I would make the formula in this strength.

Formula

Licorice - 20%

Garlic - 15%

Echinacea - 15%

Aniseed - 30%

Fennel - 20%

Look these herbs up in the herbal and consider why I used them, there are three obvious ones for Licorice alone with the first being to force the assimilation of the formula into the body, second is its expectorant action and third is its demulcent action in case the throat is sore and raw. Next time you see a little kid eating heaps of licorice get them to open their mouth and look at their tongue which will be going black from the Licorice along with the throat etc. and know that you are looking at the demulcent action of Licorice working by coating and soothing. The most important reason that you use the Actions Method for Herbal Prescribing is so that you can concentrate the Actions which are most needed for example, if it's a Bacterial Infection concentrate on the Anti Bacterials, if it's a Viral infection concentrate on the Anti Virals, hopefully you are now beginning to see the importance of working in actions for if you don't concentrate a large part of the battle on the causes you may have lost the battle from the start. Read through all the Actions listed in Herbal Actions in the book and then do a study in depth of at least five Actions of your choice making the first two the Anti Bacterials and Anti Virals. Start trying to train your mind into thinking in Actions.

How To Make Herbal Tinctures

Tinctures are made by steeping the Herb plant material in a mixture of alcohol and water. Alcohol is usually always used at strength of 45%. The alcohol in this mixture will extract all the essential oils from the herb while the water will extract all that is water soluble, so between the both we are getting most of the medicinal properties out of the herb. The proportions of herb to liquid are usually 1 part herb to 5 parts liquid. So find a suitable container (I use a big one liter preserving jar with a good sealing lid) and put into it 100grams of your chosen herb and to that add 500mls of our 45% solution of alcohol. Seal the lid and shake well for about a minute. Leave the jar on the window sill so the sun can shine on the jar for two weeks. The jar must be shaken for at least a minute every day. After 2 weeks open and filter the contents of the jar. I use a large pouring jug into which I place a funnel and then place a coffee filter in the funnel and pour the jar contents through the funnel being careful not to let too much herb spill into the filter and block it up. When you get to the bottom of the jar you can crush the herb in your fist so as to extract the last of the liquid. After this is completed you then get your chosen storage bottle, put a funnel into its neck followed by a coffee filter and then filter the jug into the bottle. Remember the solution should always be double filtered Next we label the bottle, put the date, name and proportions e.g. 1 to 5 also state the recommended dose. Store in a cool and dark place. Most Professional Homoeopaths and Herbalists have access to pure alcohol so for them it is fairly easy to make tinctures while for the lay person they will probably have a hard time. An alternative is to use Vodka as strong as you can find it or find a way to twist the authorities arm into giving alcohol at 45%. Don't even try to get pure alcohol as it is dangerous and can turn people blind and they won't give it to you.

How To Make Infusions

Infusions are a bit like making a cup of tea except we don't use milk. Infusions are used for the soft parts of the herb such as the flowers, leaves and fine twigs. The proportions for infusions are 1 to 20 e.g. 1 part herb to 20 parts water. Infusions are used for the more water soluble herbs. Infusions can be made from a single herb or from a combination of herbs and may be drunk hot or cold. The water should be just off the boil before being poured on the herb and if you are making an infusion of a herb strong in essential oils such as Peppermint always cover the top of the cup to stop the essential oils from escaping in steam while the infusion is brewing. Allow up to 10 minutes to brew. It is best to make herbal teas fresh each day. You can experiment on yourself by getting Chamomile and Peppermint tea bags from the supermarket. Use honey as a sweetener.

How To Make Decoctions

Decoctions are used for the more hard woody substances of the herb such as barks, berries or roots. The process of decoction is far more vigorous then infusion as it involves heating the plant material in cold water, bringing it to the boil and simmering for 20 to 40 minutes. The finished ratio for decoctions is again 1 part herb to 20 parts water; remember to add more water at the beginning so you wind up with the 1 to 20 after steam loss. This form of preparation is no good for the herbs that are high in essential oils as these will all be lost in the steam.

Glossary of Herbal Terms And Index Of Actions

Adaptogen - Helps the body overcome its problems and work to the best of its ability. Good convalescent herbs.

Herbs - Panax Ginseng, Siberian Ginseng .Schizandra, Withania.

Alterative - Herbs that gradually restore proper function to the body, they increase health and vitality. They were once known as the blood cleansers.

Herbs - Beth root, Black cohosh, Damiana, Dong Quai , Red Clover, Sarsaparilla, Skullcap.

Analgesic - Herbs that reduce pain.

Herbs - Black Haw, Chamomile, Dong Quai, Hops, Ladys Mantle, Passion Flower, St Johns Wort, Skullcap, Valerian, Wild Yam, Withania.

Antidepressive - Damiana, Rosemary, Skullcap , St Johns Wort, Valerian, Vervain.

Anti-fungal - Calendula, Cats Claw, Pau D' Arco, Myrrh, Olive Leaf.

Anti-inflammatory - Helps the body to combat inflammations. Herbs mentioned under demulcents, emollients and vulnerary's will often act in this way especially when they are applied externally.

Herbs - Black Cohosh, Blue Cohosh, Chamomile, Feverfew, Ginger, Ladys Mantle, St Johns Wort, Sage, Wild Yam, Withania.

Anti-microbial - Helps the body destroy or resist

pathogenic micro-organisms.

Herbs - Aniseed, Rosemary, Sage, Thyme Yarrow

Anti-oxidant - Milk Thistle, Schizandra.

Antispasmodic - Prevents or eases spasms and cramps.

Herbs - Aniseed, Angelica, Black Haw, Beth root, Black cohosh, Blue Cohosh, Chamomile, Cramp Bark, Dong Quai, Hops, Motherwort, Passion Flower, Red Clover, Rosemary, Sage, Skullcap, St johns Wort, Valerian, Vervain, Wild Yam.

Anti-viral - St Johns Wort

Antirheumatic - Black cohosh, blue cohosh, dandelion, sarsaparilla,

Aperient - Mild laxative.

Herbs -Dandelion, Fenugreek, Milk Thistle.

Astringent - Contracts tissue which in turn reduces discharges, these herbs contain tannins.

Herbs - Black Haw, Beth root, Hops, Ladys Mantle, Sage, raspberry, Rosemary, Squaw Vine, Shepherds Purse, St Johns Wort, Yarrow.

Bitter - Herbs that taste bitter act as stimulating tonics for the digestive system.

Herbs - Feverfew, Hops,

Carminative - Stimulates peristalsis of the digestive system and relaxes the stomach and helps remove gas and wind from the system. These herbs are usually rich in volatile oils.

Herbs - Aniseed, angelica, chamomile, garlic, ginger, sage, rosemary, valerian.

Cardioactive - Has a effect on the heart.

Herbs - Motherwort,

Circulatory Stimulant - Siberian Ginseng, ginger, rosemary

Cholagogue - Stimulates the release of bile from the gallbladder which can relieve gallbladder problems, bile is also the body's natural laxative so cholagogues have a laxative effect as well.

Herbs - Dandelion, milk thistle.

Demulcent - Soothes and protects irritated or inflamed internal tissues.

Herbs - fenugreek, licorice, milk thistle, sarsaparilla

Diaphoretic - Aids the skin in the elimination of toxins and produces sweat thus reducing the temperature of fevers.

Herbs - Angelica, black cohosh, chamomile, garlic, ginger, sarsaparilla, thyme, vervain, yarrow.

Diuretic - Increases the secretion and elimination of urine.

Herbs - Agrimony, angelica, dandelion leaves, false unicorn root, ladys mantle, shepherds purse, red clover, sarsaparilla, yarrow.

Emmenagogue - Stimulates and normalizes the menstrual flow, tonics for the female reproductive system.

Herbs - Angelica, black cohosh, blue cosh, chamomile, cramp bark, dong quai, false unicorn root, fenugreek, ginger, ladys mantle, motherwort, raspberry, sage, rosemary, shepherds purse, St Johns

Wort, thyme, Valerian, vervain, yarrow.

Expectorant - Supports the body in the removal of excess mucous from the respiratory system and helps in the control of coughs.

Herbs -Angelica, aniseed, fenugreek, garlic, red clover, thyme, vervain.

Febrifuge - Helps the body to bring down fevers.

Herbs - Raspberry, sage, thyme, vervain.

Galactagogue - Helps increase the flow of milk in females.

Herbs - Aniseed, fenugreek, milk thistle, raspberry, vervain.

Hepatic - Tones and strengthens the liver, may increase the flow of bile.

Herbs - Agrimony, dandelion, motherwort, milk thistle, vervain, yarrow.

Hormone Precursors - Provide the building blocks for hormones.

Herbs - Beth root, Black Cohosh, Blue Cohosh, Licorice, Fenugreek, Ginseng, Sarsparillia, Wild Yam, Withania

Infusion - Is like how you make a cup of tea but when you make herb teas you don't use milk. Pour boiling water onto the herb in the cup and cover the cup (to stop the essential oils from evaporating) and leave for about 5 minutes. To sweeten add honey.

Laxative - Promotes the evacuation of the bowels.

Herbs - Dandelion, fenugreek,

Lotion - A water and tincture mixture, example 2 parts tincture to 20 parts water.

Nervine - Has a beneficial effect on the nervous system, acts like a tonic to this system.

Herbs - Black cohosh, blue cohosh, chamomile, cramp bark, damiana, hops, motherwort, oats, rosemary, skullcap, St Johns Wort, schizandra, thyme, valerian, vervain.

Parasiticide - Kills parasites and insects.

Herbs - Aniseed, rosemary.

Pectoral - Has a general strengthening and healing effect on the respiratory system.

Herbs - Aniseed, garlic, hyssop, vervain.

Sedative - Calms the nervous system and reduces stress and nervousness throughout the body.

Herbs - Black Haw, Black cohosh, chamomile, cramp bark, hops, motherwort, passion flower, skullcap, St Johns Wort, schizandra, valerian, vervain.

Stimulants - Quicken and enliven the physiological function of the body.

Herbs - Dandelion, garlic, rosemary, sage, yarrow.

Tincture - Herbal tinctures are made from herbs mixed with a water and alcohol mix of about half and half and are usually of the strength of 1 part herb to 5 parts solvent.

Tonics - Strengthen and enliven specific organs or the whole body.

Herbs - Aniseed, Beth root, black cohosh, blue cohosh, chamomile, dandelion, fenugreek, motherwort, oats, raspberry, sarsaparilla, skullcap, thyme, vervain, yarrow.

Urinary Antiseptic - Angelica, damiana, shepherds purse, yarrow

Vasodilator - Black cohosh, Dong quai, feverfew, ginger, yarrow

Herbs Used For Females

Below are listed some of the main herbs for Female conditions that Herbalists use. Herbalists never prescribe for just the disease alone but always prescribe on an individual basis because the reality is that there is just about as many different forms of disease as there are people who have it. Some of the herbs listed below may be hard for you to find but most Health Shops and some Chemists should be able to supply it in tea form. Another place to look is at the herb section in the Supermarket where you would be able to buy the Sage and Rosemary.

With complex Herbal treatment it is best to get this done professionally making sure of course that you bring along your chart with you. The reason for this is that an herbalist will treat you holistically and not just the most bothersome symptoms. This is very important and the best way to show you is to give you an example of how I might treat someone with menopause problems.

When I make a Herbal formula which is usually in tincture form I try to use no more than 5 herbs and for a women with menopause problems one herb would go to help the liver which now has the extra job of converting androgen to estrogen and another herb (Hormone Precursor Herbs) would go to help the adrenal glands which are now doing the main job of making estrogen especially in a person who is under a lot of stress physically or mentally for this can burn out the Adrenal Glands. My remaining herbs would go to helping the main symptoms of the case but with these I would try to choose herbs that could be converted into hormones easily. So as you can now see there is a lot more that goes into it then just prescribing herbs for the symptoms.

For most people reading this you will probably make your combination of herbs in teas. As this book has been designed for people in the country away from easily accessible Medical Treatment I will go into detail about selecting and individualizing an herbal formula suitable for you.

The best way to start is to sit down and write out your main symptoms or the ones most annoying to you in order of their importance but do not go over about 8 strong symptoms for the idea is to try and keep this reasonably easy. As you have read before we try to use only 5 herbs in the formula with one being for the liver and another from our list of Hormone Precursors in the Herbal Actions List. The last 3 herbs along with the first 2 should cover most of our symptoms and for the strong symptoms we want at least the actions of 2 herbs to cover that symptom so as to enhance the action in that area. A good example is below.

<u>**Formula List of 5 Symptoms in order of Importance.**</u>

Black Cohosh	Rheumatism
Dandelion	Liver and fluid retention
Sage	. Hot Flashes
Skullcap	Insomnia, Depression
Passion Flower	Moody

Black Cohosh - (Hormone Precursor) covers the symptoms of Rheumatism and Hot Flashes.

Dandelion - (Liver Herb) covers the symptoms of Rheumatism.

Sage covers the Hot Flashes and probable sweating which is a main symptom.

Skullcap covers depression, insomnia and moods.

Passion Flower covers insomnia, moods and touches on the depression and could help with the pains of rheumatism.

The above is a good example of overlapping Actions of Herbs while at the same time having our Liver Herb and Hormone Precursor Herb. Look up the herbs individually in the herbal and take not of their Actions.

Some Useful Formulas

Here are two different formulas, one which can be taken in the morning and another which can be taken in the evening. The evening formula is designed for sleep and to help with night sweats. The formulas that follow are fairly common ones that you would probably come across in your own research. Have a look also at the ones you can buy in the chemists and try to see what they are doing with their formulas. Remember you want a tailor made formula made to you.

Morning Formula
Phyto-oestrogenic Herbs
Aniseed - A good digestive herb, antispasmodic.
Black Cohosh - One of the main menopause herbs, is a good anti rheumatic herb as well.
Licorice - Anti-inflammatory, general tonic, (don't use if you have blood pressure problems).

To these add two or one more of your own, a couple of examples are
Non Phyto-oestrogen Herbs
St Johns Wort - Depression, Anxiety, Nerve Pains, Shingles etc
Cramp Bark - For Cramping Pains.
Buchu - Urinary tract infections.

Why not add a piece of Linda's Hormone Cake.

Evening Formula
Phyto-oestrogenic Herbs
Fennel - A good digestive and respiratory herb
Hops - Sedative and digestive bitter.
Red Clover - Relaxant, good for coughs and skin problems

Sage - Antiseptic, good for sweating and hot flushes.

To these add two or one more of your own, a couple of examples are
Hawthorn - Lowers blood pressure, looks after blood vessels.
Schisandra - Liver tonic, helps with night sweats
Valerian – Sedative
Zizyphus – For sleep and hot flushes.

These are good and effective herbs and we covered a lot them when we went through the Menopause Symptoms In Detail.

These Are Some Other Menopause Formulas

Made Using herbal Tinctures
2 Parts Licorice
2 Parts Dandelion Root
1 Part Motherwort
1 Part False Unicorn Root
1 Part Wild Yam
Dose is 1 to 3 droppers of tincture to a little water.
Take 2 to 3 times a day 3 to 5 days a week.

Dr Herons Menopause Mixture
Made Using herbal Tinctures
2 Parts Chaste Tree
1 Part Motherwort

1 Part False Unicorn Root
1 Part Dong Quai
1 to 2 Parts Sage
1 Part St Johns Wort
1 to 2 Parts Black Cohosh
1 Part Licorice
1 Part Black Haw
1 Part alfa alfa
Blend the tinctures together in a bottle. Take half to one tea spoon full, mix with water 3 times a day on a empty tummy.

Rosemary Gladstars Formula
Made Using herbal Tinctures
2 Parts Wild Yam
1 Part Sarsaparilla
2 Parts Siberian Ginseng
1 Part Dong Quai
3 Parts Sage
3 Parts Licorice
3 Parts Dandelion Root
Mix the tincture in a separate bottle. Dose is a quarter of a teaspoon full 3 times daily.

Amanda's Menopause Tea
90g Chaste Tree
60g Dong Quai
30g Siberian Ginseng or Licorice
60G St Johns Wort

60g Horsetail
90g Motherwort
Mix the herbs together well. Infuse 30g of herbal
blend in 1.1 liters of boiling water, cover and steep for
20 minutes, then strain. Dose is 1 cup 3 times daily

Herbal Menopause Formulas

Below is a list of some common Menopause
Formulas found usually in boxes at your local
Chemist or Health Shop. I will give you the Brand
name first followed by the Product Name and then
will give you a list of the ingredients. It is now up to
you to look up the ingredients in the Herbal and
find which product covers most of your symptoms
and would be the most suitable for you. A lot of
these are not made any more and some of the brands
are gone but it gives you an idea of the herbs used
in some of the formulas which you can look up and
see how they work. Red Clover is a fairly common
main ingredient but with this herb all they have
done is extracted the estrogens and concentrated
them and are not using the herb for its traditional
use.

Blackmores

Dong Quai,Vitex Agnus Castus (Chaste Tree)

Good Health

Femone Herbal Relief Tablets - Soya Bean, Red
Clover, Wild Yam, Dong Quai, Black Cohosh, St Johns

Wort, Calcium.

Nutralife
Phyto Femme - Soy Extract, Red Clover, Wild Yam, Dong Quai, Vitex.

Natures Own
Menopro - Red Clover

Natural Nutrition
Menopause - Black Cohosh, Damiana, Soy, Calcium, Vit D, Magnesium.
Dong Quai Complex - Dong Quai, Black Cohosh, Wild Yam, Cramp Bark, Ginger.
Natural Womens Phase - Black Cohosh, Dong Quai, Wild Yam, Sarsparillia, Siberian Ginseng, St Johns Wort, Sage, Ginger.

Naturopathica
Meno-eze - Black Cohosh, Chaste Tree, Dong Ouai, Horse Chestnut, Licorice, Red Clover, Wild Yam, Soy isoflavones.

Natures Sunshine
Black Cohosh.
Chamomile
Damiana
Milk Thistle

Red Clocer
Sage
Wild Yam.

Novogen

<u>Rimostil</u> - Red Clover
<u>Promensil</u> - Red Clover.

Remifemin - Black Cohosh

Herbal

Aniseed

Actions - Antispasmodic, carminative, expectorant, parasiticide, antimicrobial, galactagogue.

This is a herb with many uses, some of the main uses are intestinal colic and flatulence, a good digestive tonic and appetite stimulant, a good expectorant and along with its antispasmodic action it can be used for such conditions as bronchitis and whooping cough. Aniseed has mild estrogenic effects and can be used as a good herb for relieving some of the symptoms of menopause.

This herb has a reputation of increasing milk production in nursing mothers, promoting menstruation and also facilitating childbirth. It is also said to increase libido in men and women.

Doses - Mainly used as a tea, 1 to 2 teaspoonful's of seeds add boiling water, cover and leave for 5 to 10 minutes.

Angelica

Actions - Carminative, antispasmodic, expectorant, diuretic, diaphoretic, emmenagogue.

As an expectorant it is good for respiratory infections with coughs accompanied with fever, as a digestive it stimulates appetite and is good for colic and flatulence and this herb may also be used as a urinary antiseptic in cases of cystitis. This herb is a close relation to Dong Quai which is Chinese Angelica and would have similar actions

Doses - Tincture 2 to 5mls 3 times daily, 1 teaspoon full of the cut root in tea 3 times daily.

Astragalus

Actions - Immune-modulator, anti-viral, adaptogen, hypotensive, immune stimulant, adrenal tonic, diuretic, vasodilator, blood tonic.

Stimulates the natural production of interferon (helps to stop viruses replicating) and intensifies the white cell destruction of germs in other words it is a immune booster. A good tonic for strengthening the resistance to disease. Is very useful for people in a state of chronic debility and fatigue by restoring the immune function and giving them energy especially in those with cancer undergoing chemo or people with Ross River Fever this is why the herb is known as a Adaptogen because it helps people adapt and have the energy to cope with changes. Use as a lung tonic to help expel toxins and pus in flu's, colds and sinusitis. Increases stamina and can accelerate wound healing.

Uses - Boosting immune system, disease preventative, fatigue, healing wounds, good for use in those with chronic diseases that cause immune problems such as AIDS.

Beth Root

Actions - Uterine tonic, astringent, expectorant, antispasmodic alterative.

Contains natural precursors of the female sex hormones. Is a tonic for the uterus and its astringent power is used for excessive bleeding or hemorrhage. It is considered a specific for excessive blood loss during menopausal changes. It is mainly used for bleeding due to menses, fibroids and postpartum difficulties.

Black Haw

Actions - Astringent, antispasmodic, sedative, hypotensive, analgesic, uterine tonic.

Has a similar action to cramp bark to which it is closely related. Powerful relaxant of the uterus used for cramps and false labor pains. Can be used to prevent miscarriages. It can relax peripheral blood vessels thus reducing blood pressure. Its use for bleeding is confined to birthing and menopause.

Black Cohosh

Actions - Emmenagogue, anti-spasmodic, nervine, alterative, sedative, tonic, vasodilator.

Black Cohosh has a normalizing action on the balance of female sex hormones and may be safely used to regain normal hormonal activity that should give relief to Menopause and PMS symptoms. This would be the herb for you if you also suffered from rheumatism or arthritis. Has hormone balancing properties, encourages estrogen production, painful or delayed menstruation, ovarian cramps or cramping pain in the womb, used to regain normal hormone activity, good for hot flashes, rheumatoid and osteoarthritis, muscular and neuralgic pains with a good example being Sciatica. Black Cohosh may also lower blood pressure, lower cholesterol, help with insomnia and help with tinnitus.

Doses - For tincture is 2-4mls 3 times a day, One and a half teaspoonful's for tea 3 times a day.

Cautions - Best taken with meals so as to avoid any chance of upsetting tummy. Allow up to 8 weeks to see benefits in menopausal problems and even then the full benefit of the herb may not be reached till 6 month's time. Antibiotics can reduce the effect of this herb. This herb can interfere with hormonal medications eg The Pill. Contra indicated in pregnancy.

Blue Cohosh

Actions - Nervine, antispasmodic, uterine tonic, diuretic, emmenagogue, antirheumatic.

As a emmenagogue this herb can be used to bring on delayed or suppressed menstruation while ensuring that the pain sometimes accompanied is relieved. Good for most pains and spasms associated with the menstrual cycle and reproductive organs. Can be used for leucorrhoea and vaginitis. Blue Cohosh may be used where there is a need for a antispasmodic such as in colic, asthma and nervous coughs and it also has a good reputation for easing rheumatic pain.

Doses - Tincture 1 to 2mls 3 times daily, 1 teaspoon of dried root for tea 3 times a day.

Caution - Can further increase blood pressure in people with high blood pressure.

Chamomile

Actions - Antispasmodic, nervine, carminative, anti-inflammatory, analgesic, antiseptic, allergies.

An excellent gentle sedative with a relaxing action that is good for easing anxiety and helping with sleep. In the digestive system it can be used for indigestion especially when there is colicky pains and is ideal for colitis and IBS type problems. For females Chamomile is good for amenorrhea, spasmodic dysmenorrhea, premenstrual irritability and menopausal tensions. This herb is also a good source of calcium and magnesium.

Doses - Tincture 2 to 4mls 3 times daily, for teas just the one teabag.

Cramp Bark

Actions - Nervine, sedative, astringent, antispasmodic, tonic, emmenagogue, dysmenorrhea.

As the name suggests this herb is a relaxer of muscular tension and spasms. It has to main areas of use with the first being muscular cramps and the second in ovarian and uterine muscle problems. Cramp Bark relaxes the uterus and relieves spasms and cramps and can be used to help prevent a miscarriage. This herb also has a astringent action which gives it a role in the treatment of excessive blood loss in periods and especially bleeding associated with menopause.

Doses - Tincture 4 to 8mls 3 times a day, for tea 2 teaspoonful's of the dried bark 3 times a day.

Dandelion

Actions - Diuretic, cholagogue, antirheumatic, laxative, tonic.

Here we will mainly be using Dandelion for its diuretic action so as to ease fluid retention.

For this it is best to use the leaf. Dandelion is a gentle and safe diuretic because unlike others it actually gives the body more potassium then it takes out.

Doses - Tincture 5 to 10mls 3 times daily, 2 to 3 teaspoons of herb for tea 3 times daily.

Damiana

Actions - Nerve Tonic, antidepressant (sexual matters), urinary antiseptic, alterative, reproductive tonic.

A good herb for strengthening the nervous system and it also has a tonic action on the hormonal system. Considered to be a specific in cases of anxiety and depression where there is a sexual factor. Damiana may help to reduce hot flashes and may increase sex drive and can be used for cystitis, headaches and insomnia.

Doses - Tincture 1 to 2mls 3 times daily, 1 teaspoon of dried leaves 3 times daily.

Note - Longer use of Damiana increases its potency and helps to regulate sex hormones in women but it may also interfere with iron absorption.

Dong Quai see also Angelica

Actions - Emmenagogue, antispasmodic, analgesic, alterative, uterine tonic ,vasodilator.

Relieves some but not all of the symptoms of PMS and menopause by its action as a known regulator for the female reproductive system. Some of its compounds stimulate the uterus while others relax the uterus. The compounds that stimulate the uterus are water soluble and are absorbed into the body from teas and capsules. The compounds that relax the uterus are soluble in alcohol and are provided by tinctures. This herb may stop cramping, migraine attacks and eases the pain of ovarian cysts while there is less agreement on whether the herb stops hot flashes (wait and see after 6 weeks on the herb). The Chinese use this herb for abnormal menstruation, suppressed flow, painful or difficult menstruation. This herb is also good for the treatment of psoriasis. Dong Quai also helps with Anemia related to menses, asthma, bronchitis, emphysema and improves the function of the lungs.

Dose - 6 to 18 grams of dried root per day and in the tablet form 1500mg per day.

Note - This herb has a mild laxative effect. People who take blood thinners should avoid this herb.

Echinacea

Actions - Immune stimulant, anti-microbial, anti-inflammatory, alterative, healing.

Is an infection fighter active against strep bacteria (abscesses and boils), a blood cleanser, (blood poisons, snake bites, poisonous insects) and a glandular and lymphatic system cleanser. Use it particularly for respiration infections and for any disease above the waist. This is one of our main immune boosters for the acute diseases. Use as a prophylactic to protect from infections especially when traveling or before going into Hospital.

Uses - All infections, depressed immune function, inflammatory conditions, allergies, effective against both bacteria and viruses.

Dose – 1 to 4mls of tincture

Warning - Do not use continually as you will burn out the immune system give a few weeks break after 3 weeks. Beware also in the use of allergies for you could be building up the immune system just to attack itself.

False Unicorn Root

Actions - Uterine tonic, emmenagogue, diuretic, emetic, antiseptic, vermafuge.

A tonic that strengthens the reproductive system. Contains estrogen precursors. Useful in delayed or absent menstruation, Good for easing ovarian pain, used as a aid to getting pregnant and staying pregnant as well as for vomiting during pregnancy. Can be used as a restorative tonic after long use of the birth control pill. Can help with physical and emotional wound after sexual abuse and be given to women as a tonic after menopause or hysterectomy.

Feverfew

Actions - Anti-inflammatory, vasodilator, relaxant, digestive bitter, uterine stimulant.

It is one of the most important aids for female ailments with the plant exerting remarkable powers over the uterus. A good treatment for all female irregularities especially scanty or failing menses, painful periods, inflamed or weak uterus, uterine and vaginal ulcers, abortion, difficult labour, retained afterbirth, arthritis, inflammations. May help ease dizziness and tinnitus with other remedies (Black Cohosh). Has a good reputation for migraine headaches, may help with arthritis when it is in the inflammatory stage. This herb may also help with colitis, indigestion, fevers and inflammations.

Dose - Best taken in tablet form. 3x500ml tablets a

day.

Fenugreek

Actions - Expectorant, demulcent, tonic, laxative, galactagogue, hypoglycaemic, nutritive.

This herb supports liver function and is protective to the mucous linings of the body as well as having a strong action on the lymphatic system as it clears and promotes the drainage of the body through the lymphatic system. This rubbish removing action can lead to strong body odors and dark urine and maybe even a healing crisis as a life time's load of rubbish starts to get evicted.

This is a good herd to use if you have diabetes. This herb is said to be a good hormone balancer for menopause and may raise estrogen levels.

Doses - Tincture 1 to 2mls 3 times a day, 1 and a half teaspoons of seed (crush seed first to release oils) add boiling water and cover, let stand for 10 minutes. 1 teaspoonful of aniseed can be added to improve the taste. Maybe only use this twice a day and maybe a week on and a week off.

Garlic

Actions - Immune stimulant, anti-bacterial, anti-viral, anti-fungal, anti-septic, anti-oxidant, diaphoretic, cholagogue, hypotensive, anti-spasmodic, vermifuge and many more.

The plant is rich in volatile oil and sulphur and

because of its remarkable penetrating, disinfecting and mucous expelling powers garlic is a valuable basic remedy for the treatment of all ailments in which the cleansing of the blood stream and expulsion of mucous accumulations is required. Garlic can be used to prevent and treat respiratory infections. Anyone who has had garlic breath has experienced this herb's aromatic compounds being excreted through their lungs which is why garlic's active ingredients can be so effective for respiratory complaints. Garlic is extremely effective in dissolving and cleansing cholesterol from the blood stream, it stimulates the digestive tract, kills worms, parasites and harmful bacteria, normalizes blood pressure, reduces fever, gas and cramps.

Uses- All infections, coughs, colds, flu, bronchitis, all fevers, pulmonary conditions, gastric and skin complaints, rheumatism, all worms and ringworm, ticks and lice.

Acts on Bacteria, Viruses and Internal Parasites.

Dose – 3000mg Garlic Oil tabs are the best way to go as tis gets into the blood fast. For those who cannot tolerate the breath use Kyloc the Japanese aged form as this is odourless.

Externally - You can use garlic for ring worm and ear ache, to disinfect wounds and sores, parasitical infections.

Ginger

Actions- Carminative, anti-inflammatory, vasodilator, circulatory stimulant, diaphoretic, anti-emetic.

The therapeutic benefits of ginger are largely due to its volatile oil and oleoresin content. Ginger is an excellent remedy for many digestive complaints, including nausea, colic, wind and indigestion. Its antiseptic properties also make it beneficial for gastro-intestinal infections. It stimulates the circulatory system and helps blood flow and increases stamina. Aids in fighting colds, colitis, digestive disorders, wind, and increases saliva.

Uses- Indigestion, nausea, feverish conditions especially when chills are present, travel sickness especially sea sickness, dyspepsia, colic, flatulence.

Caution - Don't use large doses on an empty stomach..

Ginseng (Panax)

Actions - Anti depressive, stimulating adrenal agent, estrogenic, increases resistance and improves mental and physical performance.

This herb can help with depression especially when caused by debility and exhaustion. It can be used in general for exhaustion and weakness. Used to increase mental and physical performance, to improve concentration, vigilance and work efficiency, stamina, for combating internal or external stress factors of any kind - athletics, endurance activities, aging, surgery, disease, infections, cold, but especially degenerative conditions and problems of old age. This is a god herb for infertility and menopause symptoms.

Doses - For the elderly and long term 400 to 800mgs per day. Short term 600 to 2000mg per day for 3 to 4 weeks then have a break for 4 weeks then you can go back on it if you wish. Remember month on month off as this herb can build up in the system. During your month off you will still be getting the benefits of this herb as the excess leaves the body.

Siberian Ginseng

Actions - Adaptogen, vaso dilator, increases stamina, circulatory stimulant.

This herb is very similar to the one above but is a milder version and can be used all the time without any breaks and does not build up in the system like Panax Ginseng.

Dose - As what is said on the packet.

Ginger

Actions - Carminative, diaphoretic, circulatory stimulant, sialagogue, vasodilator, antiemetic.

Ginger may be used as a stimulant of the peripheral circulation in cases of bad circulation, chilblains and cramp. In feverish conditions ginger acts as a diaphoretic promoting sweet and cooling the body.

As a carminative it promotes gastric secretions and is used in dyspepsia, flatulence and colic. For females ginger can be used for painful menstruation or retarded menstruation. Ginger is good to mix with any other combination of herbs because it would help the body to assimilate those herbs and increase their actions.

Doses - Dose as needed in its various forms.

Hops

Actions - Sedative, hypnotic, bitter, antiseptic, visceral antispasmodic, astringent, estrogenic.

Has a marked relaxing effect on the central nervous system and is used extensively for the treatment of insomnia. Eases tension and anxiety and may be used where this tension leads to restlessness, headaches and indigestion. This is a good herb for Mucous Colitis and colicky types of pain. According to herbal folk law elderly women who worked as hop pickers experienced a return of their menstrual cycles and other youthful attributes. This lead to the use of Hops as a hormone balancer and general restorative during and after menopause. Hops contains the most potent of all the plant estrogens.

Doses - Tincture 1 to 4mls 3 times daily, 1 teaspoon of dried flowers in tea 3 times a day or just before bed.

Ladys Mantle

Actions - Astringent, anti-inflammatory, emmenagogue, diuretic, anodyne, menopause herb.

Helps reduce pains associated with periods as well as ameliorating excessive bleeding. This herb also plays a role in easing the changes of menopause. As an emmenagogue it stimulates proper menstrual flow if there is any resistance. Because of its astringency this herb is often used in diarrhea especially in children.

Doses - Tincture 2 to 4mls 3 times daily, 2 teaspoonful's of dried herb in tea 3 times daily.

Licorice

Actions - Expectorant, demulcent, anti-inflammatory, adrenal agent, anti-spasmodic, mild laxative.

The root part is used , possessing unique pectoral and emollient properties, it is also nutritive and slightly laxative, It contains the building blocks of hormones, has a marked effect on the endocrine system, catarrh, gastric and peptic ulcers, abdominal colic. Its ability to soothe irritated mucous membranes and to break up phlegm and ease coughing sees licorice employed in respiratory conditions, coughing, bronchitis, and chest colds. Can be used for treating inflammatory and allergic conditions. Licorice has effects on the adrenal glands which are protective, restorative, tonic and stimulatory.

Uses - Treatment of cough, inflamed throat,

pneumonia, pleurisy, TB, all catarrhal conditions, gallstones, chronic constipation.

Dose – 1 to 3mls of tincture 3 times daily.

Caution - Do not use with high blood pressure. Long term use depletes potassium which raises the blood pressure. Don't use with steroids.

Milk Thistle

Actions - Cholagogue, galactagogue, demulcent.

This herb is said to rejuvenate the liver, for problems like hepatitis it is used alone at first as it drains the liver probably by its action of stimulating the gallbladder to release bile. Used to increase milk production in mothers and for gallbladder problems. The reason I put this herb here is that it is the livers job to take used hormones out of the system and if this is not happening it can lead to a lot of confusion. So make sure your liver is functioning well.

Dose - Tablets can be brought in most health shops see dosage on packet.

Motherwort

Actions - Sedative, emmenagogue, antispasmodic, cardiac tonic, nervine, reproductive tonic.

Motherwort is considered a life giving plant, beneficial for all female disorders, a general heart tonic, delayed or suppressed menses especially where anxiety or tension are involved, relaxing tonic for aiding menopause, specific for over rapid heartbeat brought on by anxiety or tension.

Doses - Tincture 1 to 4mls 3 times daily, 1 to 2 teaspoonfuls of dry herb for tea 3 times a day.

Passion Flower

Actions - Sedative, antispasmodic, anodyne, relaxant, epilepsy, shingles, asthma, hypotensive.
A good herb for insomnia and a very effective herb for nerve pains especially in conditions like shingles. This herbs focus is more on restlessness and irritability, hysteria and anxiety and is soothing to the mentally worried and overworked it acts on nervousness especially due to unrest, agitation, worry, exhaustion and cerebral excitement. Used in the treatment of convulsions, epilepsy, tremors, hypertension, nervous breakdowns, migraines and neuralgias.

Doses - Tincture 1 to 4mls 3 times daily, 1 teaspoon of dried herb in tea 3 times daily.

Raspberry

Actions - Astringent, tonic, refrigerant, parturient.
Highly tonic and cleansing improving the condition of the organism during pregnancy ensuring speedy and strong expulsion of the foetus at birth. Raspberry leaf contains ferulic acid which is a uterine relaxant that can help relieve menstrual cramps. At the same time as it relaxes the uterus itself it stimulates the

muscles that support the uterus which allows a easier menstrual flow.

As a astringent it can be used in diarrhea and leucorrhoea, it is valuable in easing mouth problems such as mouth ulcers, bleeding gums and inflammations

Doses - Tincture 2 to 4mls 3 times daily, 2 teaspoonful's of dried herb in tea 3 times daily.

Red Clover

Actions - Alterative, diuretic, eczema, expectorant, antispasmodic, bronchitis, whooping cough.

Good for treating conditions like eczema and psoriasis and other chronic skin conditions.

In the respiratory system we can use the actions of expectorant and antispasmodic to treat conditions such as bronchitis, whooping cough and maybe the eczema and asthma syndrome and as this herb seems to have a affinity for the throat we could use it for tonsillitis to. In the nervous system we can use the antispasmodic action to treat stress and nervousness along with hypertension. The alterative action of this herb helps to clean out the body and makes this herbs action on the skin very effective and it is probably this action that makes it useful in cancers especially breast and Ovary cancer. This herb is in a lot of formulas now because they extract the Isoflavones (Plant Hormones) from it and it is said to be very rich in these.

The high content of hormone in this herb was first

noted by farmers in New Zealand who noticed that sheep which grazed on Red Clover became infertile.

Doses - Tincture 2 to 6mls 3 times a day. 1 to 3 teaspoon full of dried herb in tea 3 times a day.

Rosemary

Actions - Circulatory and nerve stimulant, carminative, antispasmodic, ant depressive, cholagogue.

This herb acts as a circulatory and nerve stimulant and also has a calming and toning effect on the digestive system. These actions make this herb good for the treatment of flatulence, dyspepsia, headaches, migraines, epilepsy, vertigo, fainting, low blood pressure, asthma, coughs and colds. Recently this herb has been used to prevent breast cancer and it can help to regulate menstruation.

Doses - Tincture 1 to 2mls 3 times daily, 1 to 2 teaspoons full in tea 3 times a day.

Sage

Actions - Astringent, anti-septic, inflamed throat, tonsillitis, carminative, antispasmodic, gingivitis.

This is the classic remedy for inflammations of the mouth, throat and tonsils, its volatile oils soothing the mucous membranes. This herb can be used as a mouth wash in its tea form for treating bleeding gums, inflamed tongue, or generalized mouth inflammation, mouth ulcers, laryngitis, pharyngitis, tonsillitis and quinsy. For females this herb is soothing and regulating of hormonal problems in menopause including hot flushes and is used to reduce sweats.

Doses - Tincture 2 to 4mls 3 times daily, 2 teaspoons full of herb in tea 3 times daily.

St Johns Wort

Actions - Anti-inflammatory, astringent, sedative, nervine, antiviral, nervy shooting pains.

Has a sedative and pain reducing effect which gives it a place in the treatment of neuralgia, anxiety, tension and similar problems. Regarded as a herb to use where there are menopausal changes triggering irritability and anxiety. This herb is useful for minor depression and should not be used in cases of major depression.

Doses - Tincture 1 to 4mls 3 times a day, 1 to 2 teaspoons full of dried herb in tea 3 times daily.

Schizandra

Actions - Immune stimulant, adaptogen, Nervine, antioxidant, liver tonic, restorative, cerebral tonic.

This herb is mainly focused on the liver and is used for under function and damage to this organ along with other herbs such as Milk thistle. The reason Schizandra is included in the herbal section is because it also improves mental, physical and sensory performance and helps in the handling of stress and increases stamina. This herb can also help with night sweats and improve a poor memory and is good for the treatment of depression.

Dose - 1500mg to 8000mg per day.

Sarsaparilla

Actions - Alterative, diuretic, diaphoretic, demulcent, anti-rheumatic.

Has chemicals and properties that aid in the production of testosterone, eliminates poisons and toxins from the blood and helps clean the system, useful in scaling skin conditions such as psoriasis, used in rheumatism and arthritis. Can be used for PMS problems and for menopause as well especially for loss of interest in sex. Mixed with Penny Royal it can help to relieve hot flashes.

Doses - Tincture take to 2mls 3 times a day, 1 to 2 teaspoonful's of root in tea 3 times daily.

Shepherds Purse

Actions - Uterine stimulant, astringent, diuretic, urinary antiseptic.

Possesses important astringent properties as well as being a gentle diuretic. It has a specific use in the stimulation of the menstrual process while also being used to reduce excess flow or any other type of bleeding condition in the area. Organ remedy for kidneys and bladder, tonic to pelvic organs.

Doses - Tincture 1 to 2mls 3 times a day, 1 to 2 teaspoonful of dried herb in tea 3 times a day.

Skullcap

Actions - Nerve tonic, sedative, antispasmodic, stress, anxiety, PMS, antidepressive, alterative.

Skullcap has a wide range of use mostly focusing on the nerves. It relaxes states of nervous tension while at the same time renewing and revivifying the central nervous system. It has a specific use in the treatment of seizure, epilepsy and hysterical states. It may be used in all exhausted or depressed conditions. Good for easing Pre Menstrual Tension and painful menstruation.

Doses - Tincture 2 to 4mls 3 times a day, 1 to 2 teaspoonful's of dried herb in tea 3 times a day.

Squaw Vine

Actions - Astringent, nerve tonic, diuretic, emmenagogue, restorative, dysmenorrhoea, parturient

This herb can be taken for the relief of painful periods, amenorrhea, menorrhagia, uterine bleeding and chronic congestion of the uterus. Squaw Vine is more well known for preparing the body for child birth and helping with complications after birth.

Doses - Tincture 1 to 2mls 3 times a day, 1 teaspoonful of herb in tea 3 times a day.

Valerian

Actions - Sedative, hypnotic, antispasmodic, hypotensive, anxiety, PMS, antidepressive.

One of the most relaxing nervines available that can be used to safely reduce tension and anxiety and is also a very effective herb for chronic insomnia. As a antispasmodic it will give relief to any cramp like and colicky pains and is a good pain reliever in general helping with rheumatic and migraine pains. Can also be used for nervous exhaustion and high blood pressure.

Doses - Tincture 2 to 4mls 3 times daily. 1 to 2 teaspoons full of root in tea 3 times daily.

Vervain

Actions - Nerve tonic, sedative, antispasmodic, diaphoretic, hepatic, antidepressive, hypnotic.

This herb is a combination of a Nervine and a Hepatic so it can be used to treat doth systems. As a Nervine it can be used for stress, tension and as a general relaxant and it is also used to ease depression and melancholia especially after illness or influenza. As a hepatic it has been found to be of help for problems such as inflammation of the gallbladder and jaundice. This herb may be of some help in migraine headaches.

Doses - Tincture 2 to 4mls 3 times a day. 1 to 3 teaspoonful's of dried herb in tea 3 times daily.

Vitex Agnus Castus (Chaste Tree)

Actions - Hormone balancer, progesterone precursors, PMS, menopause.

This herb has a stimulating and normalizing effect on the pituitary glands functions especially its progesterone function. The main use of this herb is for normalizing the activity of female hormones and is indicated for dysmenorrhea, PMS, Menopause and is also used to help restore balance for female going of birth control pills. Other uses are Acne and Endometriosis.

Doses - Tincture 1 to 2mls 3 times a day, 1 teaspoonful of the ripe berries in tea 3 times a day.

Note - This herb may take a month or 2 to start working and when it does start working it is necessary to take the herb for 3 to 6 months after symptoms disappear.

Yarrow

Actions - Astringent, digestive, diuretic, antiseptic, peripheral vaso dilator, menstrual regulator.

A good herb for fevers and for lowering blood pressure. As a antiseptic diuretic Yarrow is good for the treatment of cystitis and is also used to regulate menstruation at puberty and menopause.

Doses - Tincture 2 to 4mls 3 times a day. 1 to 2 teaspoonful's of dried herb for tea 3 times a day.

Wild Yam

Actions - Antispasmodic, anti-inflammatory, ovary and uterine pains, visceral relaxant, colic.

This herb was once the sole source of the chemicals that were used in the early contraceptive pill. The antispasmodic action makes it valuable for the relief of colic and menstrual cramps and dysmenorrhea along with ovarian and uterine pains. Good for nervy type pains.

Doses - Tincture 2 to 4mls 3 times a day, 1 to 2 teaspoonful's in tea 3 times a day.

Withania (Ashwagandha)

Actions - Adaptogen, analgesic, anti-tumor, hormone regulator, pregnancy tonic, rejuvinative.

This herb is a pregnancy tonic for both the foetus and a weak mother, relieves pain by lowering serotonin levels which contribute to the sensitivity of pain receptors in the body. Good for debility, nervous exhaustion especially due to stress and chronic diseases especially those marked by inflammation. Retards various aspects of the aging process and increases stamina and also sexual desire.

Doses - As on packet.

Zizyphus

This is the new kid on the block that is being used in a

lot of the new menopause formulas and also sleeping remedies. This herb has been used in Chinese medicine for over 4000 years. One write up I read said. The seed is used in TCM to quieten the spirit, for dream disturbed sleep, insomnia, irritability, palpations with anxiety and spontaneous night sweats.

Homeopathic Supplement

Homeopathy has been around now for hundreds of years and unlike most other forms of medicine its rules have not changed and will not for they are based on an essential truth. The main rule is Like cures Like or if we break down the word Homeopathy homo means the same and pathy means disease. As Homoeopathy is a very hard science to learn and as it kind of sits or balances on the border of hard science and metaphysics I will not try to explain to you what it is here as it would probably take a whole book to do this but I will say this, in the UK and a lot of countries in Europe it is on and paid for by the National Health System and anything that can get a politician to open their purse must work.

It is said that Homeopathy sits on a three legged stool. What this means is that if a remedy has at least three symptoms in the same strength as the symptoms you are trying to match then that remedy is a potential cure for your condition or if not cure it will offer the condition relief. The more symptoms you can match to the remedy the better the remedy will work for the rule is likes cure likes not vaguely similar cures. Listed below are some common Homoeopathic Remedies and some of the symptoms they cover. The idea is to find one remedy that covers most of your symptoms. To make the remedies as closer a match as we can we ask lots of questions like the ones below and after we gather all the answers we have what is called a good Symptom Picture which we then try to match as accurately as we can to a Remedy. Most Homeopathic Materia Medicas are set out to answer the questions listed below with the mind symptoms being the most important. Questions on time, position and temperature are good for making a choice between to very close remedies. The best Materia Medica for the lay person is Boerickes and you should be able to view this on a few Homeopathic websites.

Symptom Guide Questions

1/. Was there a sudden onset of the condition, at what time?

2/. What time of the day does the patient feel either better or worse.

3/. What is the effect of motion? jarring? walking? running?

4/. What is the effect of drinking fluids? warm and or cold drinks?

5/. Is the patient thirsty or not at all? sips or gulps?

6/. Is the onset from exertion? overeating? weather changes? emotions?

7/. Mental emotional state of patient?

8/. Better warm room? warm air?

9/. Better cool room? cool open air?

10/.Are the respirations upper chest movements or in the abdomen?

11/.Respirations - dry or wet?

12/.Expectoration - watery or stringy mucous, easy or difficult.

13 Is there coughing

14/. Position - better or worse from sitting? standing? lying? lying on which side?

15/. Along with the condition is there fever? gas? belching? wind?

Modality - The questions above are covering what the Homoeopaths call modalities which basically mean are covering a condition that makes the patient better or worse. I will list the main Modalities below. The Modalities help us to distinguish which remedy is right for the case especially when we have a group that look as though they may all work which is what I am giving you und the disease heading. Using modalities forces you to think what really is going on, is this the nature of the beast or the nature of the disease.

Time - Better or Worse morning, night, weekly, monthly, seasonally etc.

Motion - Better or Worse first movement, rest, exertion, walking, stretching, rising up etc

Temperature - Better or Worse heat, cold, cold air blowing, sudden change etc.

Body Activity - Better or Worse eating, drinking, urinating, defecating, sleep, coughing etc

Weather - - Better or Worse, damp, sunny, foggy, storms, sudden changes etc.

Senses - Better or Worse - touch, pressure, noise, light, odors etc.

Position - Better or Worse lying, standing, sitting, stretched out, doubled up, right side etc.

Mind - Excitement, anger, fear, stress, better busy, nervous all the time etc.

Now read through all the remedies in the Marteria Medica (Homoeopathic Remedy Reference) and you will notice that most of them have Mind or mental symptoms kind of describing the personalities or moods a good example is Nux Vomica, I think we all know a nasty type of individual that this remedy would be suited to and meaning as though the individual is suited to this remedy then the remedy would have a curative action on them but don't expect it to change the nature of the beast. One of the main rules of Homeopathy is the closer the match of the remedy the higher the Potency you use but if you are not used to Homoeopathy just use the 30C potency and remember what I said about the 3 legged stool. Potency is a measure of strength and depth of action.

Remember as mentioned before Homoeopathy sits on a three legged stool. What this means is that if a remedy has at least three symptoms in the same strength as your symptoms then that remedy is a potential cure.

Note - The best prescribing guide for the layman is **Boerickes Materia Medica With Repertory.**

Another good guide is **The Complete Book Of Homeopathy by Dr Michael Weiner.**

I always buy my books on Homeopathy from India as they are quarter the price and there is always a wide selection. Put B. Jain Publishers into the google search engine go to their web site and check out these books and I am sure you will be pleased with what you find.

How To Use This Section

In the Marteria medica that follows you are given all the Homoeopathic remedies that are used in the Complexes and most of those mentioned in Cystitis. The symptoms guide gives you the knowledge of the questions to ask to find a good Homoeopathic remedy which you can use to find with the many online repertories that are available. When you have found a remedy that you think suits you look it up in Boerickes Marteria Medica as this is one of the easiest to use even though it is in old English. Below are all the remedies used in the complexes. The Estrogen 4C is a slightly different form of Homoeopathy that I kind of think of as body parts homoeopathy. Generally it works like this. A low 4C potency of Estrogen tries to stimulate the body to produce more Estrogen while a 9C potency of Estrogen makes the body think there is too much thus reducing Estrogen. This can be used for example in my PMS kit where sometimes I want to reduce a hormone as it may be leading to unwanted problems so I give it in the 9C potency with an example being Progesterone 9C to try to lower it. Now you can start to see a whole new method of controlling Hormones.

The Homoeopathic Complexes
For Menopause Kit

1. **Meno A:**   This is the main complex and is made up of Estrogen 4C, Calc Phos 6X, Nat Mur 6X, Lachesis 12C, Sepia 12C, Pulsatilla 6C

2.   **Meno B:** Covers the symptoms of depression, emotions, mood changes and headache. **It is made up of Sulphur 6C, Ignatia 6C, Cimicfuga 4X, Lycopodium 6C.**

3.   **Meno C:** Covers the symptoms of pain and cramps and is made up of Mag Phos 6X, Cimicfuga 4X, Colocynthis 6C.

4. **Meno D:** covers the symptoms of vaginal dryness, pain and incontinence and is made up of
Causticum 6C, Ferr Phos 6X, Lycopodium 6C

There are 4 Stock Bottles in the kit and they are labelled

1.   Meno A : which is the main remedy to which the others are added.

2.   Meno B : add to A for the relief of **Depression, Emotions, Mood Changes and Headaches**.

3.   Meno C : add to A for the relief of **Pains and Cramps**.

4.   Meno D : add to A for the relief of **Vaginal Pain, Dryness and Incontinence**.

Meno A : is the main remedy, for this remedy has the hormone Oestrogen in it. The other remedies can be added to

your dose to counter other symptoms as and when they occur.

Treatment Using The Kit

In the kit are 4 Homoeopathic Complexes based on the main groups of symptoms that occur with menopause. Homoeopathy has been around now for hundreds of years and unlike most other forms of medicine its rules have not changed and will not for they are an essential truth. The main rule is Like cures Like or if we break down the word Homoeopathy homo means the same and pathy means disease. As Homoeopathy is a very hard science to learn and as it kind of sits or balances on the boarder of hard science and metaphysics I will not try to explain to you what it is here as it would probably take a whole book to do this but I will say this, in the UK and a lot of countries in Europe it is on and paid for by the National Health System and anything that can get a politician to open their purse must have a lot of truth in it.

For the kit I am not using Homoeopathy in the way it was designed but am grouping together certain remedies to cover certain groups of symptoms in low potencies, hence the name Complexes.

Before using the kit you should be well on the way to sorting out your diet and you should be using the supplements that you feel you need for your appropriate symptoms as well as having made some good lifestyle changes especially on the exercise and de-stressing side.

Note - **Do not mix stock bottles together, add what you need to the dose.**

How to Take The Complexes

1. The 4 bottles are your Stock Complexes and must not be mixed together.
2. To take a dose place 15mls of pure water in your measurer cup and add 4 drops of the stock complex.
3. If you wish to make a mixture of 2 or more complexes just add the stock complex needed to the water in the measuring cup. (Never mix the stock complexes together).
4. When you have prepared what you need sip your dose slowly.
5. Do not eat, drink, smoke or clean teeth for about 15 minutes before or after taking a remedy.
6. Dosage is about 3 to 4 times daily.

Materia Medica

Note - All Homeopathic Remedies are given in Potency and not in material Form.

Aconite

Characteristics - Aconite is best used in the first stages of a illness, especially when fear and anxiety are present. Symptoms appear suddenly, without warning and they may be caused by exposure to cold winds or draughts or by a severe fright. Symptoms are a marked restlessness, displays extreme anxiety or fear, high fever with a burning skin, extreme sweating and a burning thirst, a hoarse dry painful cough, bright light noises stress and cold worsen the symptoms, rest and quiet relieves the symptoms. The pains of Aconite are unbearable, sharp, shooting, burning pains, tingling and numbness. A remedy for fevers and inflammatory states, use at the first sign of all fevers, shivering with cold sweats, difficult breathing, shows desire for large quantities of water, symptoms worse at midnight, symptoms improve in the open air. In women dry vagina. Menses to profuse, ovaries congested and painful.

Mind - Great fear, anxiety, restlessness, extreme sensitivity to pain, worry, foreboding.

Better - In open air, warmth, rest.

Worse - In the evening and night, particularly before midnight, lying on affected side.

Allium Cepa

Characteristics - Increased secretions from the eyes and nose, like those of the common cold. Frequent sneezing with watery discharge which burns the nose and upper lip, but the eye discharge is bland and doesn't burn (the opposite of Euphrasia). Tickling in the throat with incessant cough (feels as if larynx is split) holds throat when coughing. Being in cool open air relieves the symptoms, eyelids are swollen and red, abdominal tympany with wind, this remedy is indicated in the early stages of most catarrhal conditions..

Better - Cold room (except cough), open air.

Worse - Evening, warm room, odors.

Antimonium Tartaricum - Ant Tart

Characteristics - Is characterized by a loose rattling unproductive cough.. Respiration can be very difficult with much gasping. There is usually thirst for little and often. Symptoms are worse in the evening, lying down and in cold damp weather or a warm room. Confined largely to respiratory diseases, abundant bronchial secretions, great rattling of mucous with little expectoration, drowsiness, debility and sweat. Burning in urethra during and after urinating, last drops bloody with pain in the bladder, urging increased.

Mind - Drowsy and despondent, fear of being alone, child will not be touched without whining.

Better - Sitting erect, from burping and expectoration.

Worse - Evenings, lying down, damp cold weather.

Apis

Characteristics - Apis is used for various types of swelling and inflammation such as that from animal bites and bites and stings from insects, it is also used for measles, mumps, sore throats, sore red eyes and fever. Apis is a quick acting remedy for inflammations especially those ones with edema and lots of swelling which is its main use. Acute nephritis with scanty and burning urine there may be some blood in the urine. . Symptoms are swelling with edema which makes the effected parts look shiny, red and puffy, the swollen parts feel soggy and waterlogged, a fever that develops rapidly but without thirst, extreme restlessness and fidgeting, an irritable nature and perhaps jealous, cool air and cold compresses relieve the symptoms. Pains are burning and stinging, arthritis with swelling, animals seek cold surface to lie on, swollen eyelids, may be swollen ears, may be blood in the urine. Symptoms get worse from heat and improve in the open air and from cold bathing. In women edema of the vulva, inflammation of the ovaries, stinging pains, dysmenorrhea with severe ovarian pain, ovarian tumors, metritis with stingy pains, burning and soreness when urinating, incontinence.

Mind - Apathy, indifference, awkward.

Better - By cold, (room, air or application)

Worse - From warmth, pressure, late in the afternoon, from sleeping.

Arnica

Characteristics - Bruises and similar injuries where the skin is unbroken and there is mental or emotional shock. Symptoms are any type of bruising or similar injury caused by crushing, squeezing or wrenching, muscles strains which feel sore and bruised, shock after accidents, there is a fear of being touched because of the pain, good for the soreness after birth and medical operations.

Arnica can be used in potency and also as a cream. The cream must not be used on broken skin or wounds**Mind** - Fears touch or approach, whole body oversensitive.

Better - Lying down or with head low.

Worse - Least touch, motion, damp and cold.

Arsenic Album

Characteristics - Burning pains relieved by heat, anxious, restless, weak and chilly with an air of fear and hopelessness. Anxiety or restlessness are often present where this remedy is indicated. Discharge from eyes and nose are watery and acrid causing ulceration in those regions. The mouth is usually dry and the patient is usually thirsty. Dramatic vomiting and diarrhea often simultaneously indicate its use if the modalities agree. The patient may have wheezing respiration and allergic asthmatic conditions can respond well. The skin can be dry, scaly and scruffy. Symptoms are worse for cold and wet better for warmth. Tries to find relief in motion but immediately feels weak with movement. Restless, feels cold, complains of general weakness, discharges burn the skin. For women menses to profuse to soon, burning in ovarian region, leucorrhoea acrid, burning, offensive and thin, bladder as if paralyzed.

Mind - Fear with despair and restlessness.

Better - Warmth, open air, relieved by sweat, hot drinks, lying down (but restless).

Worse - Cold air, after midnight eg 1 to 3am. Wet damp weather and near sea shore.

Belladonna

Characteristics - This is one of the great fever remedies, conditions requiring its use usually being of violent and sudden onset. Heat, redness, pain and swelling characterize its symptoms. It is one of the main remedies used in convulsions. Pupils are usually dilated which is a keynote for this remedy. Acute ear inflammation where there is heat, pain and swelling respond well. The mouth is usually dry and there is great thirst. With Belladonna always think BIRDS. B for burning, I for irritability, R for redness, D for delirium and S for spasms. For women acute urinary infections, urine frequent and profuse, sensitive forcing downward, as if all the viscera would protrude at genitals, dryness and heat in vagina, menses increased bright red to early, to profuse, mastitis pain, breasts feel heavy and hard and red, tumors of breast.

Mind - Hallucinations, delirium, rages, bites, strikes, desire to escape.

Better - For quiet, dark, rest with slight warmth.

Worse - For noise, touch or jarring motion.

Bellis Perennis

Characteristics - Trauma to abdomen and pelvic organs especially after surgery and child birth if arnica does not give relief. Injuries to the nerves with intense soreness, back ache from hard physical work such as gardening, pain is bruised sore and aching, better cold presses, worse touch, after getting wet. Unwilling to move and when made to do so causes pain, muscular stiffness is prominent. In women uterus feels sore as if squeezed.

Worse - Left side and cold wind.

Bryonia

Characteristics - This remedy shows both diarrhea

and constipation symptoms, the latter usually in chronic conditions. The mouth is often dry and there is great thirst. The tongue is often coated yellow. It is of great help in many cases of rheumatism or arthritis where the symptoms agree. There is often respiratory signs with a hoarse hacking cough. All symptoms are worse for movement and better for rest. In women menses to early, to profuse, worse from motion, menses suppressed with headache, ovary pains tender to touch, pain in breasts during period, breasts hot and painful, menstrual irregularities with gastric problems.

Mind - Irritable, delirium.

Better - Lying on the painful side, pressure, rest and cold things.

Worse - Warmth, motion, morning, eating and touch.

Calendula

Characteristics - The part used is the Flowers and it is used for wounds and skin irritations, it is healing, soothing, anti-inflammatory, astringent, anti-fungal and anti-microbial.

Use as a lotion for cuts, grazes, infected sores, fungal infections, any skin inflammations, regulates the oil production of the skin so is good for acne, to stop bleeding, for bruises and sprains, skin ulcers and minor burns and scolds.

Note - The tincture of this is used as a lotion diluted

at 1 to 10.

Cantharis

Characteristics - Important first aid remedy for minor burns and for other pains that feel burning and fiery, also has a healing effect on the bladder, urethra and other parts of the urinary tract where burning pain is the key symptom, burns and scalds especially where blistering and inflammation occur, sunburn, insect bites that feel hot and burn, cystitis. Pains are violent burning, cutting, stabbing or smarting, rawness.

Mind - Furious delirium, acute mania generally of a sexual type, crying, barking.

Better - Better from warmth rest and rubbing.

Worse - From touch or approach, from urinating, from drinking cold water.

Carbo Vegetabilis

Characteristics - Patient exhibits mental and physical sluggishness and symptoms come on slowly, generalized weakness of all functions especially digestion, overweight, torpid, lazy, complaints of coldness, pains usually described as burning, pressing pains, wishes to be fanned, digestive problems such as belching often accompany any illness. In women menses copious an early, swollen vulva leucorrhoea before menses thick greenish milky and excoriating, during menses burning in hands and soles.

Mind - Aversion to darkness, sudden loss of memory.

Better - Being fanned, passing gas, rest.

Worse - Morning and evening, exertion, cold, tight clothes at abdomen.

Causticum

Characteristics - Burns and burning pains such as cystitis also used for dry coughs, burns to the skin especially with marked inflammation and blistering, coughs, laryngitis and hoarseness from straining and over using voice, cystitis especially with involuntary passing of urine when coughing, chronic cystitis, exposure to cold dry air may make symptoms worse. For women menses cease at night only flows during day.

Mind - Least thing makes it cry, sad, hopeless. Ailments from long lasting grief.

Better - In damp wet weather, warmth.

Worse - Cold winds.

Cimicfuga

Characteristics – This remedy has a wide action on the nerves and muscles. Nervous subjects with ovarian irritation and nervy pain, uterine cramps and heavy limbs. Agitation and pain indicate this remedy, pains like electric shocks here and there. Migraine symptoms. Amenorrhea, pain immediately before menses, menses always irregular. Ovarian pains, Oversensitive to pain.

Mind – Great depression and low spirits,, incessant talking.

Better – Warmth and eating

Worse – Morning, cold, during menses.

Euphrasia

Characteristics - Affects the mucous membranes of the eyes, nose and chest producing copious watery secretions, eye secretions cause smarting of the skin while the nose discharge is bland. Used for conjunctivitis, eye strain generally but especially from computers, eyes that feel sore and inflamed and look red, hay fever symptoms including a tickly throat, sneezing, a runny nose, and itchy red watering eyes. Sunlight wind and warmth worsen the symptoms. In women menses painful, flow lasts only an hour or day, amenorrhea with ophthalmia.

Better - In the dark

Worse - From light, indoors, in the evening.

Hypericum

Characteristics - Used for bruises and other injuries especially to nerve rich areas like the fingers, lips, ears, eyes ,tail bone, good for the pain of puncture wounds of any cause eg animal or insect.

Helps with the pains after operations especially amputations. Pains are violent shooting pains along a nerve path, burning, tingling and numbness. Worse from shock and touch and better from rubbing, horse fly bites, symptoms worse cold better warmth.

Mind - Anxiety, melancholy, effects of shock.

Better - Bending head backward.

Worse - Cold, dampness and touch.

Ignatia

Characteristics – Suited for the nervous. sensitive, highly conscientious, excitable people with gentle dispositions. The emotional state is of quick alternating moods. Labor like pains. Menses to profuse or scanty. Feminine sexual frigidity.

Mind – Changeable moods, introspective, silently brooding, melancholic, sad, tearful. Not commutative.

Better – Change of position, hard pressure.

Worse – Morning. Coffee, external warmth.

Ipecac

Characteristics - Indicated for complaints of persistent nausea not relieved by vomiting, ailments caused by eating rich or indigestible type of foods such as ice-cream, sweets etc., useful to stop bleeding if blood is bright red. For women uterine hemorrhage profuse bright blood gushing with nausea, pain from navel to uterus.

Mind - Easily irritated, child cries or screams continuously, wanting something but not sure what they desire, holds everything in contempt.

Worse - Warm, moist weather, lying down.

Kali Bichromicum

Characteristics - Has an affinity for the mucous membranes of the body, tough stringy viscid secretions sometimes forming thick yellow green mucous, sinus infections, suited for fleshy fat light complexioned people, general weakness.

Better - Heat

Worse - Cold, beer, morning, undressing.

Kali Carbonicum

Characteristics - Has an affinity for the mucous membranes digestive and respiratory, very tired, anemic, flabby tissues which may be swollen, sweat, backache, weakness, many conditions have an aggravation at 2am to 4am, often stays immobile when ill.For women menses early, profuse or to late pale and scanty.

Mind - Very irritable, hypersensitive to pain, despondent.

Better - During the day, sitting down, bending forward, warmth.

Worse - Cold weather, between 2am and 4am.

Lachesis

Characteristics - Many symptoms tend to be left sided, cannot bear tight clothing, symptoms worse on awakening, symptoms relieved with onset of the menstrual flow. Short dry cough, feels relief after coughing up watery phlegm, feeling of constriction in throat and chest, better bending forward. For women climacteric troubles, palpitations, flashes of heat, menses to short to feeble, all pains relieve by the flow, left ovary painful and swollen.

Mind - Overly talkative, impatient, sad, jealous, no desire to mix with world.

Better - Release of pressure, eating fruit, cold, discharges.

Worse - Pressure, touch, after sleep, heat, hot weather.

Ledum

Characteristics - Has an action on the capillaries and is useful for cleaning up bruises especially around the eyes, mainly used for puncture wounds made by sharp points such as nails and wood splinters and insect bites and stings especially ones that don't heal properly and look blue and puffy. Wounds that feel cold to the touch, septic conditions, sprains, pains are throbbing, tearing ,prickling, they shoot upwards, stiff and sore. Better cold, cold bathing. This remedy was used in the past along with hypericum to ward off tetanus especially in deep wounds

Better - From cold.

Worse - At night and from heat.

Lycopodium

Characteristics - Exerts most of its effects on the digestive organs, liver, kidneys and respiratory systems. The patient dislikes being left alone and appears apprehensive. The nose is often blocked and there may be blisters on the tongue. Eating a little food always satisfies the appetite but appetite is very marked. The belly is usually bloated. The stool appears hard and small and is expelled only with difficulty accompanied by ineffectual straining. Urination is also a slow process and the urine has a red sediment. For women vagina dry, sex painful, right ovarian pain, leucorrhoea acrid with burning in the vagina.

Mind - Melancholy, afraid to be alone, apprehensive.

Better - By motion, on getting cold.

Worse - From heat.

Natrum Sulphuricum

Characteristics - A good liver remedy, emotional and mental difficulties arising after head injury, useful in problems associated with rainy weather and dampness, patient feels every change from dry to wet weather, may remove excess water and fluid retention from the body. For women menses irregular, usually profuse, vagina dry, leucorrhoea acrid and watery.

Mind - Lively music saddens, melancholy, inability to think, dislikes to speak or be spoken to.

Better - Dry weather and environments, pressure, change of position.

Worse - Damp weather, damp basements, lying on left side.

Nux Vom

Characteristics - The remedy for overindulgence, adapted especially to thin irritable energetic people who attend with great detail to tasks, quarrelsome, nervous, intelligent, hypochondriacal, oversensitive to noise music and light, craves stimulants.

Primarily used in the digestive sphere, its greatest reputation is in helping disturbances following overeating of unsuitable foods. Feces is usually hard but diarrhea can follow overeating. There is abdominal discomfort, flatulence, irritability and sensitivity to noise. For women menses to early lasts to long, always irregular, prolapse.

Mind - Very irritable, sensitive to all impressions, malicious, disposed to reproach others.

Better - Wet weather, lying down, uninterrupted nap.

Worse - Overeating, mental over exertion, sensory

stimulation ie sound, sight, touch etc.

Phosphorus

Characteristics - Irritated and inflamed mucous and serous membranes are the key feature of this remedy. Is a very sudden remedy with suddenness of symptoms. The patient is sensitive to loud and sudden noises (eg thunder fireworks etc). Degenerative processes and bone destruction respond well to Phosphorus. Food is suddenly vomited back up when it has been warmed in the stomach, gums can be ulcerated and bloody. Hepatitis, jaundice, pancreatic disease and nephritis come into its sphere. Urine may be bloody. A very painful cough is also a symptom. Wounds that perpetually bleed may also be helped. The patient is usually in poor body condition. For women menses to early and scanty, lasts to long, leucorrhoea profuse, smarting, corrosive, instead of menses.

Mind - Low spirits, restless, fidgety.

Better - In the dark, lying on the right side, from the cold, sleep.

Worse - Touch, from exertion and in the evening.

Pulsatilla

Characteristics - Often indicated for those with mild, gentle, timid yielding dispositions who are easily moved to laughter and tears, The Pulsatilla person wants to be held and loved, moods changeable and fickle, the patient is chilly but desires strolling in cold air, symptoms are erratic and change frequently, pains are wandering, pains that grow gradually in intensity, fever without thirst despite dry mouth, bland yellow discharges. Changeable menstrual flow, starting and stopping.

Mind - Weeps easily, timid, fears to be alone - dark - ghosts, likes sympathy and fuss, highly emotional, easily discouraged, sensitive.

Better - Open air, cold applications, consolation relieves symptoms.

Worse - Evening before midnight, warmth, after eating fat rich food.

Rhus Tox

Characteristics - Is the most famous of the rheumatic remedies. The skin and muscular skeletal system are its main spheres. Small red papules in the skin and sometimes vesicles are typical lesions with much scratching. In all cases of damage to muscles think of Rhus and the symptoms of arthritis which are worse after rest particularly if this follows strenuous exertion. The symptoms improve with limbering up , The worst pains are seen as the animal arises from its bed. For women swelling with intense itching of vulva, menses early, profuse and prolomged, acrid.

Mind - Listless, sad, extreme restlessness, great apprehension at night.

Better - Warmth, walking, from stretching out limbs.

Worse - During sleep, cold wet rainy weather and at night.

Ruta

Characteristics - Has effects on the joints, tendons, cartilages, and the periosteum which is a fine membrane that covers bones and gives it that shiny look, it is also used for eye strain where the vision goes dim.

Used for painful bruises affecting the bones, dislocations, strains to the tendons or joints, aching with restlessness, pains are gnawing, digging, burning, bruised, sore as if beaten, bones as if broken, pain deep in the bones, rheumatism.

Better - From lying and warmth.

Worse - From over exertion, touch, cold wet weather.

Silica

Characteristics - Fits the shy chilly patient who is reluctant to enter the room, chronic inflammatory conditions such as sinus, helps in the removal of foreign bodies such as splinters and seeds, ripens abscesses, ailments attended with pus formation. Use silica and be prepared to use it for a while sometimes up to 3 weeks. For women leucorrhoea milky acrid, itching of vulva and vagina, discharge of blood between periods, vaginal cysts.

Mind - Faint hearted, anxious, yielding.

Better - Warmth, wet or humid weather.

Worse - Morning, from lying down, cold.

Staphysagria

Characteristics - Suits sensitive people who suppress their feelings and suffer in silence or who boil over with indignation, remedy for cuts and wounds especially those that are from medical procedures and have the mentioned feelings. Nervous states of animals. The pains are stinging, stitching, smarting, squeezing, as if stabbed by a knife. Worse from touch, emotions and suppressed anger. For women part very sensitive, worse sitting down, prolapse.

Better - Warmth, rest at night.

Worse - Touch on affected parts, loss of fluids.

Sepia

Characteristics – Often pale flabby persons with fair but flushed skin, sensitive to external influences such as touch and jarring. Exhausted dragging down sensations, better in the afternoon, wore in the morning and evening. Ailments from sexual excess. prone to problems of the sexual organs. Organs feel as if forced out through vulva, menses usually late and scant. Leucorrhoea yellow, greenish with much itching, menses to late, scanty, irregular, prolapse, vagina painful especially during sex.

Mind – Indifferent to those loved best, averse to occupation, to family. Dreads to be alone. Very sad. Weeps when telling symptoms.

Better – Afternoon and from exercise.

Worse – Morning, evening, sensory stimuli such as touch, light, noise and storms.

Symphytum

Characteristics - Causes bone to grow and promotes fast healing should be given for all fractures. Used for injuries to the hard parts of the body while arnica is for the soft parts. Also used for eye injuries caused from blows.

Caution - do not use if a pin has been placed in the bone as the pin has to be removed latter.

Tarentula Cubensis

Characteristics - For abscesses, boils, carbuncles, swellings of any kind but especially on the back of the neck where the skin turns black, red/blue or purple with great pain. Deep septic conditions with hardening of the effected part, condition comes on fast, pains are burning, stinging, throbbing, pricking like a needle.

Worse - Night.

Urtica Urens

Characteristics - Can be used for burns and also for cystitis where the urine burns the skin and there is difficulty passing urine. Symptoms are stinging pains, swellings particularly blistery swellings, itching. For women leucorrhoea acid and excoriating, uterine hemorrhage, stinging and itching of the vulva with odema, excessive swelling of the breasts.

Worse - Cool moist air, touch

What If I Need More Help

Hopefully most of your problems should be over or greatly improved if not you should have a fair idea of what's happening to you from your personal chart and some patterns should be coming apparent. Nutrition is the most important step to good health, make good use of your Acid and Alkaline Chart for this is the key to health and always take into consideration that your body is always replacing itself, the blood every 3 months, the skeleton every 12 months etc, so in a year's time are you going to have a body made of good food or a junk food body. If all else has failed the next attack will be with Herbal Remedies in the form of tinctures or teas targeted directly at your specific symptoms as well as a tonic for the liver so as to improve its function.

If after all of this you are still not happy you could go to a Doctor and show your Symptom Diary which should be fairly long by now and tell of the treatment you've had which no doubt will be ridiculed and then you would probably be offered hormone treatment and in some extreme cases surgical intervention. Never be afraid to speak your feelings and always be in control of what is done to you, don't give your power away and take the best from all worlds. Remember we must always try to remove the cause not the end results.

Estrogen Replacement Therapy (ERT)

Women with any of the following conditions should not be on ERT

A history of endometrial or breast cancer, liver disease, severe diabetes, blood clot formation, undiagnosed genital bleeding, endometriosis, fibroids, high blood pressure.

Risks Associated with ERT

Side effects of treatment may be as follows

1.   Nutrient Deficiencies - Folic Acid, Zinc, Vitamins C, B6, B2, B1, and essential fatty acids.

2.   Vaginal bleeding, weight gain, leg and pelvic pains, oedema, digestive upsets, nausea, vomiting. Increased risk of cancer of the endometrium or uterine lining.

Reducing The Risk Of ERT

1/. Use the lowest dose and shortest time possible.

2/. Stop treatment every now and again to see if you

still need it.

3/. Be examined every six months.

4/. Estrogen should be administered with progesterone (use natural progesterone not synthetic).

Last of all I want to say especially to people with severe problems don't be afraid of using Hormone Treatment that Doctors usually prescribe for severe problems as this form of treatment can bring reasonably fast relief and you can use this treatment to get yourself over the worst of the problems then slowly wean yourself off as your health improves. Problems with hormone replacement therapy seem only to happen to the long time users but if you use it just to get yourself over the worst and improve your health while you are doing this and keep on using your chart you should come out alright at the end.

Disclaimer

The information in this booklet is given as a General Guide and the author accepts no responsibility for self-treatment and advices that if you are in doubt seek Professional Help.

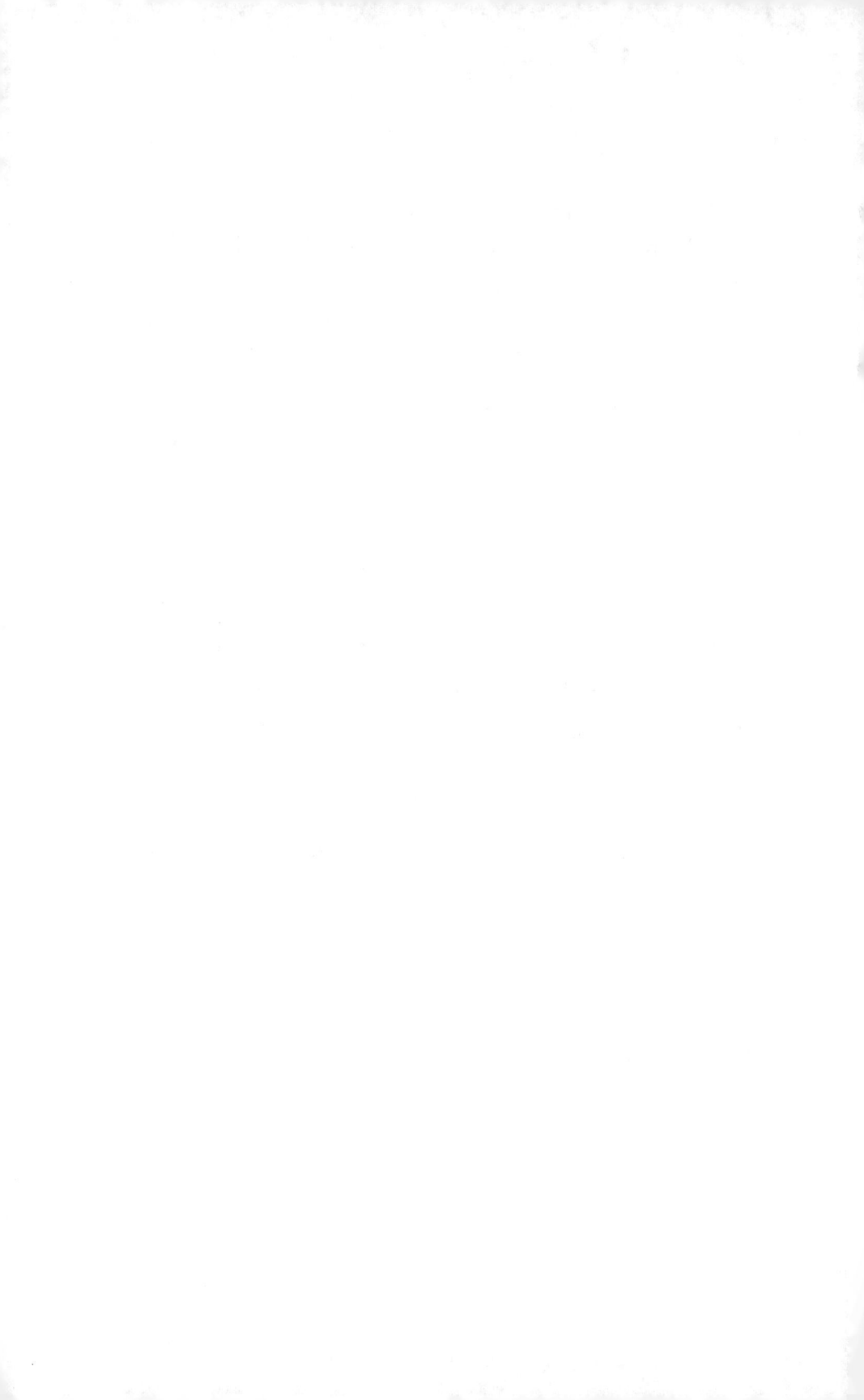

www.ingramcontent.com/pod-product-compliance
Lightning Source LLC
Chambersburg PA
CBHW051516170526
45165CB00002B/489